Living with HIV

by Michael Carter

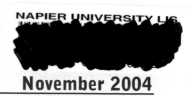

November 2004

NAM, Lincoln House, 1 Brixton Road, London, SW9 6DE

Living with HIV
First edition, November 2004

ISBN
1 898597 59 7

Copyright ©
NAM 2004

Data conversion
Thomas Paterson

Production
Joe Kaler

Cover design
Alexander Boxill

Printed in the UK by
Unwin Brothers, Surrey

With the financial support of:

PETER MOORES FOUNDATION

also:
Gavin Hay, Lyndhurst Settlement, Thomas Sivewright Catto Charitable Settlement, The Body Shop Foundation

Special thanks to:
Paul Bateman, James Chalmers, Susan Cole, Stephen Edwards, Caroline Guinness, Dr Mark Nelson, Carolyn Partrick, Nick Partridge, Positive Nation, Positively Women and all my colleagues at NAM

NAM contact details:
email: info@nam.org.uk   tel: 020 7840 0050   fax: 020 7735 5351   website: http://www.aidsmap.com

NAM — for HIV information

NAM was founded by Peter Scott in 1987. He was working at the heart of the community affected by HIV - at the London Lesbian and Gay Switchboard. At that time it was important to produce a clear, plain language resource in the face of extensive misinformation about HIV and AIDS, much of it confused and homophobic.

NAM now also publishes a wide range of printed, audio and electronic materials for all communities of people with HIV and publishes on the internet at www.aidsmap.com. The work is rooted in the experiences of those most affected by the epidemic.

NAM believes information enables people to take control of their lives and healthcare, develop better dialogues with their healthcare staff and so live longer, healthier lives.

Preface

The first guide to survival written by people living with AIDS in the UK was published in 1987. Looking at "Living with AIDS" now and comparing it to "Living with HIV 2004" shows both how much has changed and how much we still have in common with those writing 17 years ago.

Many of the personal issues remain - coming to terms with your diagnosis, who to tell, looking after yourself, sex life, employment, coping with fear, illness and going into hospital. But the emphasis is wholly different. In 1987, preparing for the future included making a will and considering the kind of funeral you would want. Now, for many people, it's about staying in work and planning for a pension.

"Living with AIDS" was just 20 pages long, mentioned only two anti-HIV drugs and yet was optimistic about research and the future. For many, that optimistic future has arrived. So we now need to understand things like viral load and CD4 counts, combinations of 18 drugs in four classes with more to come - as well as getting on with life.

Like its predecessors, this book comes directly from the experience of people living with HIV. It pools and shares information, knowledge and insight, which has always been the foundation for taking control of any illness. For anyone living with HIV, this guide will be invaluable.

Nick Partridge
Chief Executive
Terrence Higgins Trust

Contents

Contents cont.

Introduction – Living with HIV

Introduction

This book is for people who are HIV-positive. It's hoped that it will contain something useful both for people who have been recently diagnosed with HIV and for those who have known that they have HIV for some time. It's been written with a UK readership in mind.

The book includes information on the medical and social aspects of life with HIV and aims to provide basic answers to some of the questions you may find yourself asking. You might want to read the book cover-to-cover, or just dip into it at times when you need to find something out.

The information in this book isn't exhaustive, and it isn't intended to replace discussions with your doctor or any other professional. But it should provide an introduction to the key issues involved in living with HIV and help you decide what further questions you may need to ask.

NAM produces a range of HIV information books, booklets and leaflets, and some of these are listed at the end of each chapter as suggestions for further reading.

Included in the book are first-hand accounts written by people who are living with HIV. They're not meant to be examples of what you should do, they just give an idea of how people have coped with the realities of day-to-day life with HIV. Thanks to everybody who sent contributions. Every effort was made to include them all, but there simply wasn't room. Sorry if yours wasn't included.

The last time NAM produced a book of this kind, called *Living with HIV and AIDS* (which was a successor to the 1987 Frontliners' publication, *Living with AIDS*), was in early 1996, just before effective anti-HIV treatments became available. Since then, the use of combinations of anti-HIV drugs has brought about incredible improvements in the health and life expectancy of people with HIV. This book takes account of this turn-around in the fortunes of so many people living with HIV, but also acknowledges the real problems still involved in life with HIV.

Information from NAM's *AIDS Reference Manual*, including the chapters on travel, HIV and the law and hepatitis have been adapted for inclusion in this book.

Thanks to everybody who was involved in the preparation of *Living with HIV and AIDS* and the *AIDS Reference Manual*. Your hard work has made the preparation of this book very much easier than it would otherwise have been.

Life on HAART – a personal perspective by Michael Carter

For the past six years I've been taking antiretroviral therapy. I've seen my CD4 cell count quadruple and my viral load fall from the high hundred thousands to below 50 and stay there. It would be easy to conclude that, for me, the treatments have been a success – not least because it's over 13 years since I was diagnosed with HIV and 11 years since my first AIDS-defining illness. To put it simply, without anti-HIV drugs I expect I would be dead now.

However, I am still very much aware of the seriousness of HIV, of the extent to which it impacts on my life and of the fact that it is likely to continue to do so for the foreseeable future.

I'm still very medicalised. I go to the HIV clinic every eight weeks for blood tests to monitor the success of my treatment and its impact on my metabolism. This means I see my consultant just as often as I did before I started taking anti-HIV drugs.

Living with HIV has also had an impact on my mental health – just as the lab results began to suggest that the damage it was doing to my immune system was being controlled, my mental health declined. I've had two major depressions since I started HIV treatment, each of them as debilitating in their own way as any physical illness HIV has caused me. Both my consultant and the specialist HIV psychiatrist he referred me to have assured me that I'm far from alone in experiencing mental health problems after starting treatment. For some, these are direct side-effects of their medication. For me, the causes have been less direct. I've had periods of real pessimism, and the renewed hope for the future which treatment has given me has been compromised by side-effects and uncertainty.

Fortunately, I've been spared any of the disfiguring changes in body shape (lipodystrophy) which some anti-HIV treatments can cause. A friend, however, has not been so lucky, and has developed severe facial wasting which has required several courses of treatment to correct even temporarily. As he put it: "It's the ultimate irony – you're spared dying of AIDS only to look as if you are."

I've had my fair share of side-effects as well, including the diarrhoea that accompanied my first year on nelfinavir, which felt like a tap being turned on in my bowels. Then there was the peripheral neuropathy in my feet and lower legs – the worst pain I've ever been in, which still isn't completely resolved, five years after stopping the drug which caused it. At one point I had to see a cardiologist, after I developed an irregular heart beat. As I've no obvious risk factors for heart disease – indeed, I've run three marathons in the last year or so and am training for a fourth – the increased blood fats which some anti-HIV drugs can cause looked like a possible cause. Thankfully it turned out to be nothing more worrying than the consequence of having a low resting heart rate, from all the running I do. But it required numerous visits to the hospital, and I still ask my doctor about my cholesterol levels with some concern.

When I'm feeling optimistic, I can well envisage anti-HIV treatment keeping me well and living to a ripe old age. But every time I have my viral load measured, I worry that it may have become detectable again. I'm only human, and despite my best efforts I occasionally miss taking a dose of my treatment or take it a few hours late.

There's also uncertainty about how long my body can tolerate infection with a chronic viral illness like HIV and the potent drugs needed to treat it. I'm more than aware of the excess rates of certain cancers seen in people with HIV, and, as I've had warts in my anus and rectum in the past, I'm particularly concerned by reports that even when anti-HIV drugs are working well, people with HIV who've had anal warts have an increased risk of anal cancer.

Coupled with the medical uncertainty is a lack of security, particularly as regards money. Although I've managed to stay in the same job for over two years now, HIV meant that I had a very chequered employment history for over a decade. I'm now in my late 30s, and don't own my own home (and doubt that I ever will). I've started paying into a personal pension plan, but worry that I've left it too late. I really do worry that chronic poverty could be awaiting me in old age – if HIV treatment keeps me alive that long.

But there's a need for a bit of perspective. I'm not the only person I know who worries about money and security. It's far too easy to blame HIV and treatment side-effects for just about every medical condition that raises its head. For example, I noticed a slight thinning in my cheeks recently, and my instincts were to attribute this to treatment-associated fat loss rather than to look at a less sinister explanation, like the fact I'm fast approaching 40.

With treatment has also come a redefinition in the way I perceive myself and, I think, the way others look at me. I've no doubt that I'll live a longer and healthier life thanks to antiretroviral therapy. This means I'm starting to expect things from life – not least enjoyment and fulfillment. I'm no longer prepared to accept the day-to-day drudge that accompanied my pre-treatment days with HIV. Nor, if another drug option exists, do I see why I should have to cope with side-effects. I've become bored of hiding my HIV status – if somebody asks me how I got a housing association flat with a garden in central London I now tell them, "because I have AIDS." It normally stops any further questioning. Nor do I worry about looks or enquiries when I take my pills in public.

But there are still limitations to my honesty and openness. I've never told my parents I have HIV. As they are aging and I'm very well, I now doubt that I ever will. I'm lucky that I've never had a bad reaction from anyone I've told I was HIV-positive. Okay, a few Americans on gaydar seemed to lose interest when I told them – but then if they want to rely on people knowing their own status, and revealing it, as their method of avoiding infection, then more fool them.

But despite my best efforts, popular prejudice about HIV has penetrated deep into my consciousness. I do feel guilty that the medical services provided for my treatment are so good when my chronically ill parents have to wait months for appointments and even longer for treatment and care.

Thanks to the success of treatment, I no longer feel that people should make the allowances for me which they were prepared to make in the past. I'm very aware of how hard it's been for my partner and friends at times. The problems I'm facing now are less serious, and are more generic – a lot of people have controllable chronic illnesses; a lot of people live with pain; a lot of people are financially insecure.

I want to make the most of the fact that HIV treatment means that I'm alive when I expected to be dead. But I also need to acknowledge that life with HIV medication brings its own set of problems. Like HIV itself, they've become part of my life, and, with varying degrees of success, I've had to find ways of coping with them.

Just found out you're HIV-positive?

Introduction

Being diagnosed with HIV will be one of the most significant events in your life. It's very difficult to predict exactly what emotions and feelings you'll experience in the first few hours and days after finding out you have HIV, as these vary so widely from individual to individual. However, commonly reported reactions include feeling numb, frightened, upset, tearful, desperate or angry. Although it should be noted that other people have said they were relieved to have finally found out, or even excited.

It might be difficult to appreciate this at the time, but finding out that you are HIV-positive puts you in a position where you can start to take steps to look after your health. Although there's no cure for HIV and it can still be fatal, there are treatments which mean that people with HIV can live much longer and healthier lives. The sooner your HIV infection is diagnosed, the sooner you can receive appropriate medical care.

The fact that you have HIV might be the only information you can absorb on the day of your diagnosis. You should have had post-test counselling after you received your test result, and you may have been able to ask a few questions at this stage. There are no right or wrong questions to ask, and don't worry if you didn't understand everything you were told. There'll be opportunities to get more information later.

Finding out the basics

It's perfectly okay to want the most basic information, such as, 'What's the difference between HIV and AIDS?' Or, 'How long before HIV makes me ill?' Or, 'Will HIV kill me?' The first chapter of this book, 'HIV, the basics', should answer your questions.

You may also come across lots of medical terms you don't understand. Always ask your doctor, a nurse or a pharmacist to explain anything you don't understand, and ask for written information if you still have questions or uncertainties. If you want more detailed information on a particular topic, the chances are that there'll be a chapter in this book focusing on the subject you're interested in.

Getting HIV treatment and care

You are going to need specialist medical care for your HIV. Most people in this country are tested for HIV at sexual health clinics (although some people are diagnosed through other medical services), which usually have a specialist HIV clinic attached. The doctor, nurse or counsellor who gave you your test result should have made a follow-up appointment for you to see a specialist HIV doctor. If this wasn't arranged, you need to make sure that you are registered with a specialist HIV clinic as soon as possible. There's information on this in the chapter *Getting HIV treatment and care*.

If you are well at the time of your HIV diagnosis, you'll probably need to go to the clinic for a check-up every three months or so. At your appointment with your doctor you'll have an opportunity to discuss your health and ask questions, and you will have some blood tests to monitor your health.

Finding out about tests

There are two key blood tests used to assess the impact HIV is having on your immune system. These are called CD4 cell counts and viral load tests. A CD4 cell count gives a rough idea of how healthy your immune system is, and the viral load test gives an indication of how active HIV is in your body. The more active HIV is, the lower your CD4 cell count becomes, and the greater your risk of becoming unwell because of HIV. Find out more about these tests by reading the chapter *Key tests to monitor HIV*.

Making decisions

Immediately after your diagnosis can be a difficult time to make major decisions. These decisions might include who to tell about your HIV diagnosis or when to start anti-HIV treatment.

It's highly unlikely that you will have been asked to start taking anti-HIV treatment the day you found out that you were HIV-positive. It's more likely that your health will be monitored, so both you and your doctor can understand how your body is coping with HIV. If your immune system has already been weakened by HIV, then the decision to start taking anti-HIV drugs to prevent you getting the infections and illnesses to which HIV can make you vulnerable will be a more pressing one. But anti-HIV treatment is something that you will need to consider sooner or later. You can find out when you need to start treatment, what medicines you need to take, how often you need to take your medicines and what side-effects you might experience in this book.

Take time to think about who you are going to tell that you are HIV-positive. Think about why you want to tell them and how you are going to tell them. Can you anticipate their best or worst reactions? Begin by telling the people closest to you, who will be the most supportive. This book includes a chapter, *Telling people you are HIV-positive.* which provides more information on telling people in all sorts of situations.

You're not alone

There's a lot of professional support available to you. In the weeks and months after your diagnosis, you might find that counselling helps you work out your reactions to having HIV.

There are two helplines which you might find particularly useful at this time, both of which can provide basic information on HIV and are staffed by trained counsellors who will help you talk through some of your feelings.

These helplines are:

• THT Direct on 0845 122 1200.

And

• National Sexual Health Helpline on 0800 567 123

Knowing that you're not the only person going through your experiences might also be helpful, and some people find that meeting other HIV-positive people helps them to overcome their own feelings of stigma about having HIV. Some HIV organisations have events for the recently diagnosed. Don't feel that you have to attend a group if you're not comfortable with the idea, and don't think you've made a mistake if you've reacted to your diagnosis differently to the way somebody else has. There's no right or wrong way to respond to finding out you have HIV – the important thing is that you start to get information and medical care so that you can stay healthy and live as long as possible. This book should provide a useful first step.

Further reading

NAM factsheet, *Recently diagnosed.*

'Introduction to HIV and AIDS,' in NAM's *HIV and AIDS Treatment Directory.*

I've just been told I'm HIV-positive, leaflet produced by the Terrence Higgins Trust.

Lorraine's story

I was diagnosed HIV-positive five and a half years ago. My husband had been ill for the previous 18 months, but not with anything they could put a name to. It was only when he went into hospital for tests to find out why he was literally wasting away that they found out he had pneumonia. More tests revealed it was PCP.

The night he told me that he was HIV-positive, I was relieved, which was a funny reaction. I thought that at least we had a name to his illness and he could be treated. Later on, I thought about myself and whether I was infected. We were both under the impression that I would be fine, as I looked and felt really healthy. But then the GP rang me the next night...

The following weeks passed in a daze. My husband developed an infection, which, combined with working and looking after our two children, meant nothing sank in.

I knew nothing about HIV, but not through complacency – I had seen the government advertising campaigns in the late 1980s, but I had been married for 18 years. Now, I had so many questions, so many fears. The emotions I experienced were so complex I couldn't put them into words. I could just about cope from minute to minute.

Meanwhile, my husband made a partial recovery but was given only weeks to live. I left my work to focus on keeping the family together for however long we had. A few months later, things had sunk in, and I contacted the George House Trust in Manchester. There I met the most wonderful, inspiring group of women. With their support, strength and experiences, I began to feel human again. Unfortunately, my husband died the following year. A few months later, combination therapy became available and suddenly there was hope.

When I was first diagnosed, the only thing I wanted was to speak to another woman who had gone through the same thing. So when I saw the position for regional coordinator advertised, I applied. I thought that if I could be of help to anyone I would, in a way, be giving back all the support I had received.

We have a very good support group in Manchester, and doing my voluntary work has made me realise how lucky I was to have that support. There are many women around the country who are isolated – through fear of being 'found out', through not knowing who to contact, because they are carers or mothers or because they have no transport or facilities nearby. That is why this work is important – I can be just a voice on the telephone, a point of contact as and when it is required or I can arrange to meet up with them, one to one. Then perhaps, when they are ready, I can introduce them to local support services. Everyone is different and their circumstances and needs change, but no one should go through it alone.

This testimony first appeared on the website of Positively Women, www.positivelywomen.org.uk. Thanks to both the writer and Positively Women for giving permission to reprint it here.

HIV, the basics

HIV

HIV stands for human immunodeficiency virus. It was identified in the early 1980s, and belongs to a group of viruses called retroviruses.

HIV prevents the body's immune system from working properly. Normally, the immune system would fight off an infection, but HIV infects key cells in the body's natural defences called CD4 cells, which co-ordinate the body's response to infection. Many CD4 cells are killed by being infected, and others, including some cells that remain uninfected, stop working properly.

AIDS

Over time, the gradual weakening of the immune system leaves the body vulnerable to serious infections and cancers which it would normally be able to fight off. These are called 'opportunistic infections' because they take the opportunity of the body's weakened immunity to take hold.

If you develop certain opportunistic infections, you are diagnosed as having AIDS. AIDS stands for Acquired Immune Deficiency Syndrome. Different people diagnosed as having AIDS may become unwell with different illnesses, depending on the specific opportunistic infections they develop. This is why AIDS is not considered a disease, but a syndrome – a collection of different signs and symptoms, all caused by the same virus, HIV.

HIV transmission

HIV is present in the blood, semen and vaginal fluids of infected people, and can only be passed on to another person if these fluids get into his or her body. Although HIV has been found in the saliva of some people with HIV using very sensitive laboratory equipment, it is in such small quantities that it is not infectious.

The main ways HIV is transmitted are:

- By anal or vaginal sex without a condom. HIV cannot pass through good-quality condoms, and the failure rate of properly used condoms is extremely low.

- Through blood-to-blood contact. This mainly happens through sharing infected drug injecting equipment. In the past, before screening was introduced, some people were infected with blood and blood products during medical treatment. Very rarely, healthcare workers have been infected after accidently pricking themselves with a needle contaminated with HIV-infected blood.

- From a mother to her baby. This is also called vertical transmission, and can happen during pregnancy, birth or breastfeeding.

Detailed information on HIV transmission can be found in the sections on *Sex and HIV* and *Mother-to-baby transmission of HIV*.

The HIV test

HIV infection is normally detected using an HIV antibody test. This test looks for the antibodies the immune system produces to fight HIV infection. It is now very accurate.

The overwhelming majority of people infected with HIV will produce antibodies within 45 days of infection. Some people produce antibodies sooner, and in a very small number of people it can take six months, or even longer, for antibodies to appear after infection.

The HIV antibody test is not an 'AIDS test.' There is no such thing.

Tests can also be used to look for HIV itself (an antigen test) or parts of its genetic material (a PCR – polymerase chain reaction – test), often called a viral load test. Viral load testing is covered in a lot more detail in the section *Key tests to monitor HIV – CD4 and viral load.*

Stages of HIV infection

Becoming HIV antibody positive – seroconversion

Some people have a short illness soon after infection, called a 'seroconversion illness' because it coincides with the period during which the body first produces antibodies to HIV. Common symptoms include a fever lasting more than a few days, aching limbs, a blotchy red rash, headache, diarrhoea and mouth ulcers.

The severity of symptoms can vary considerably between people – they can be so mild as to go unnoticed or so severe that admission to hospital is required. It's now thought that the longer and more severe the symptoms, the greater your chance of developing AIDS within five years, presuming that you do not take anti-HIV drugs.

Doctors are currently trying to see if taking anti-HIV treatment soon after you are infected with HIV is of any long-term benefit. You can find out more and about HIV treatments in the section *Anti-HIV treatment.*

HIV infection without symptoms

Initially, any effects which HIV is having on the immune system don't cause outward signs or symptoms. For this reason, this period is called 'asymptomatic HIV infection' and it can last for months or several years.

But even if you are feeling 100% well, HIV might be damaging your immune system. Doctors use two key laboratory tests to see how active HIV is and what impact it is having on your immune system. These tests are a CD4 cell count, which gives a rough indication of the strength of the immune system, and an HIV viral load test, which shows how active HIV is in the body. Both these tests are discussed in a lot more detail in the section *Key tests to monitor HIV – CD4 and viral load*.

Sometimes you may notice that your glands, or lymph nodes, in various parts of your body become and stay swollen. This is called PGL, or Persistent Generalised Lymphadenopathy. This can happen when you've no other symptoms, and isn't a sign that you are becoming unwell or are at increased risk of doing so in the near future.

HIV infection with symptoms

The longer you live with HIV without treatment, then the greater your risk of developing symptoms. These can be caused by infections that take advantage of your weakened immunity, certain cancers and/or the direct effects that HIV can have on the body.

An AIDS diagnosis

If you have certain serious infections or cancers which have been confirmed by tests, then you will be diagnosed as having AIDS. In the US, if your CD4 cell count falls to below 200, the level at which you become vulnerable to serious infections, you are also diagnosed as having AIDS.

More than a definition

A model for describing HIV progression has developed to suggest that there is an inevitable, one-way course in HIV infection. It implies that everybody with HIV will be initially well, then get abnormal CD4 and viral load tests before becoming ill with minor illnesses, and finally go on to develop severe and fatal illness.

This has been the pattern for many people, but others have had very different experiences. For example, some people have had an illness which has led to them being diagnosed with AIDS, and then completely recovered and lived for many years, even decades, in very good health. What's more, many people who have had HIV for many years have never experienced any illness or disease because of HIV.

HIV treatments – the changed reality of living with HIV

The continuous development of new and improved medical treatment both for HIV and the illnesses it can cause has led to major changes in the pattern of HIV disease progression which people in the UK and other rich countries can expect to experience.

First of all, doctors became very skilled at treating some AIDS-defining illnesses. For example, the pneumonia PCP was often fatal in the very early days of the HIV epidemic. Now, doctors are able to control it, and people who have had it go on to live healthy lives for many years afterwards.

What's more, doctors know how to prevent many infections from occurring in the first place. Once your immune system becomes damaged to such an extent that you are vulnerable to certain infections, it is possible to take medicines to prevent these developing. This is called prophylaxis. It's considered in more detail in the section *Symptoms and illnesses*.

However, the biggest improvement of all came in the mid-1990s, when effective treatment that targets HIV itself became available. These antiretroviral treatment have led to very substantial reductions in the numbers of people dying of HIV or becoming ill because of HIV in this and similar countries. Use of antiretroviral drugs has been shown to prevent peoples' immune systems from becoming weakened by HIV. What's more, antiretroviral therapy has also been shown to work for many people with advanced HIV disease, including people with AIDS, for many of whom anti-HIV drugs have brought about a remarkable recovery in health.

Treatments for HIV are considered in a lot more detail in the chapter *Anti-HIV treatment.*

Prognosis

The prognosis for people with HIV has changed dramatically since the first cases of AIDS were diagnosed in the early 1980s. In those early days, it was thought that most people would die within a few months of first being diagnosed with the condition. This changed, partly because it was recognised that HIV was the cause of AIDS and that it took many years to gradually destroy the immune system, and partly because doctors gradually learnt more about recognising and treating infections and cancers commonly seen in people with HIV. By the mid-1990s (before the introduction of effective anti-HIV treatment), it was thought that in rich countries such as the UK it would take between eight and fifteen years (on average) after infection with the virus for HIV to cause life-threatening illness or death.

Many HIV doctors now believe that provided a person with HIV receives effective anti-HIV treatment before their immune system has been severely damaged by the virus, and if they take their drugs properly and can tolerate them, they could live a more or less normal life span.

The use of Highly Active Antiretroviral Therapy (HAART; combinations of drugs which slow down the rate at which HIV is able to reproduce) from the mid-1990s onwards has led to dramatic improvements in the prognosis for people with HIV. For instance, AIDS deaths in the UK have fallen from a peak of over 1,500 in 1994 to approximately 400 a year at present. The AIDS deaths which still occur in this country often involve people who are diagnosed with HIV late in the disease process, when their immune system is already severely damaged.

Research into the prognosis of people starting HAART indicates that the risk of becoming very ill or dying because of HIV within the next three years is linked to five key factors: having a CD4 count below 200 or a viral load above 100,000 at the time of starting treatment; being aged over 50; being an injecting drug user; or having had a prior AIDS-defining illness.

In the UK it is recommended that anti-HIV treatment is started before your CD4 count falls below 200, which is an indication that HIV has damaged your immune system to such an extent that you are vulnerable to serious illness. It is also strongly recommended that you start anti-HIV drugs if you become ill because of HIV. Starting treatment in these circumstances has been shown to improve prognosis compared to delaying treatment until later.

You can find out more about when to start HIV treatments in the section *Anti-HIV treatment*.

Some non-AIDS-related illnesses are seen relatively frequently in people with HIV, despite the effectiveness of HAART. These include liver disease caused by hepatitis viruses B or C; certain cancers, such as lung cancer, testicular cancer and anal cancer; and mental illnesses such as depression. In addition, HIV treatments themselves can cause long-term side-effects which can seriously affect health or quality of life.

There's more information on hepatitis B and C in the section on *Symptoms and illnesses*, and depression is considered in a lot more detail in the section on *Mental health*. The section *Side-effects* provides a lot more information about these.

Obviously, there are many other causes of ill health apart from HIV, and so more general health advice (such as stopping smoking, taking regular exercise, eating a balanced diet) is also relevant to people with HIV. To find out more about these issues, read the section *Daily health issues*.

Further reading

NAM factsheets, *Infectiousness, HIV's lifecycle* and *Prognosis.*

'Introduction to HIV and AIDS,' in NAM's *HIV and AIDS Treatment Directory.*

So how does HIV affect my body?, leaflet produced by the Terrence Higgins Trust.

Not just a label

I was told I had HIV in the spring of 1991, was told I had symptomatic HIV disease a year later, and received an AIDS diagnosis in the summer of 1994 after developing tuberculosis. I thought I was on a one-way road leading to an early death caused by an AIDS-defining illness.

It hasn't quite worked out like that. Although it seemed so significant at the time, my AIDS diagnosis is now pretty meaningless.

My current CD4 cell count is about 1000, my viral load is undetectable, and I'm the right weight for my height. I've no doubt that this is largely due to the success of my anti-HIV combination, which I've been taking since summer 1998.

I had a few side-effects, but have had no major physical health problems since starting anti-HIV drugs. It's no exaggeration to say that I'm one of the healthiest people I know – and that includes all my HIV-negative friends!

So, useful as my official AIDS diagnosis might be for government figures, it's pretty meaningless to me. All it does is remind me of the extent to which anti-HIV treatment has improved my health and given me the chance to get on with my life again.

The bus of doom, by Caroline Guinness

I've recently read the *His Dark Materials* trilogy by Philip Pullman (which, if you haven't already read, I highly recommend). In this theological novel disguised as a children's book, a group of kids are pursued through parallel universes.

I was struck by the concept, as we have recently moved from London to rural Wiltshire, and the contrast between the two is obvious. I grew up on a farm in Cape Town and had wanted to get out of London for many years, as I feel so much more at home in the country.

But quite aside from my daughter being at school in London and having all her friends there, I was too nervous to stray far from my HIV clinic.

Once I did fall seriously ill, while staying with friends near here. Rather than face the local A&E, I got into my car and drove 200 miles to the Royal Free in north London. I promptly passed out in the waiting room and on coming to was asked how I got there. I said that I had driven from Dorset. They gasped. "But Caroline, you have a temperature of 104 and E-coli septicaemia!" "Yes," I answered, "That's why I drove here."

But now I've had six years of successful HAART, married a fabulous man, and my daughter is at university in America. So I thought it was time to take the plunge and go back to my country roots. Through a friend, we found a gorgeous 400-year-old thatched house on a country estate near Salisbury, and four weeks ago we moved in. I promptly forgot about HIV, and telling the locals about it seems not so much impossible as irrelevant. I will drive up every three months for the usual check-up at my clinic and catch up with friends at the same time, but almost instantly I felt the stress fall away. Our two dogs and cat think they have landed up in paradise. We do not need to drive to the nearest park for a walk – it is right outside our front door.

Everything was perfect until my daughter returned for a break, and we decided to drive to London so she could catch up with friends. Setting off on a sunny day, we got to a crossroads just outside the nearest village, where there is a completely blind corner. I edged the car out so I could look to my left and was promptly hit by a bus driving at around 60 miles an hour.

It all happened in a second. I blacked out for a few minutes and came round to find the airbags in our faces and smoke pouring out of the car. How we stepped out alive I don't know. The car was a complete write-off and the bus missed my daughter by inches.

Other than a few bruises, we seemed to be physically OK, but the shock was indescribable. In the midst of it all, however, I found myself laughing. In all the years of having HIV, the one thing that drove me completely mad was the old phrase: "Yes, but everyone dies one day. You never know, you could be hit by a bus!"

I would try to explain that being diagnosed with a terminal illness was very different, and anyway, how many people did they know who had ever actually been hit by a bus?

Well, I have now. Here I am, 16 years after diagnosis, eleven years past the sell-by date I was originally given, still alive, still HIV-positive, but no longer in a position to feel anger at one particular unthinking remark. Next time someone mentions being hit by that bus I'll say, "Well, I already have, actually."

I am now getting country sympathy about the appalling driving of the local bus drivers, speed limits on country roads and how this corner has been a notorious black spot for years. Also the odd condescending remark, such as, " Oh well, now you know that driving is different here in the country. You'll have to adjust." Parallel universes, indeed. Takes the mind off HIV, anyway.

This first appeared in issue 80/81 of Positive Nation, July/August 2002. Many thanks to both Caroline and Positive Nation for giving permission to reprint it here.

20 years and counting

I became infected in 1984 and this month celebrated the fact that not only was it my 51st birthday, but also I had survived twenty years. On the weekend of my 31st birthday I received an unwanted gift, which unfortunately could not be taken back and exchanged for vouchers. I have thus spent the major portion of my adult life with the virus underlying almost every decision and action. Prognosis for me in early 1985 was that "another six months" was unlikely and that I should ensure that "my affairs were in order".

I have survived, I believe, through a combination of factors; good luck probably being the most relevant. I have been enormously lucky for the unconditional acceptance and love that I have received from my family and friends and the depth and quality of medical support that I have been privileged to obtain. I've worked hard at it as well; not prepared to give up in what is simply an instinctive fight for survival.

Nobody needs telling that life ain't easy. Fear, depression and loneliness were almost constant companions, but there were lots of good times too. I got into a very intimate and enduring relationship with alcohol, from which I have eventually managed to extract myself. Life and some degree of sanity somehow survived that affair, but it was a very close call at times.

Telling people you are HIV-positive

Don't rush

Telling people that you have HIV can seem like a daunting or even frightening task. It's important to think about who you are going to tell, and your motivation for telling them. Don't rush into telling people – although you can tell people you have HIV later, you cannot un-tell somebody.

On first learning that you have HIV, or later, when you perhaps receive bad test results, you may feel a desire to unburden yourself and tell somebody. However, you may regret this later. Although you might want people to know what you are going through at times like this so you can receive their support, there are other times when you might find this intrusive – you may not want to be asked constant questions about your health, how you are feeling or how you are coping. It might even seem that you are having to support and reassure the people who you told about your HIV.

We all react to difficult and stressful situations in different ways. Similarly, there's no rule of thumb about what sort of support you should ask those close to you to provide. Think about what's best for you. The most important thing is that you feel you have control over who you tell about your HIV.

Practicalities

If you decide to tell somebody that you have HIV, think carefully about what you are going to tell them, and how, where and when you are going to do this. Also think about how they are going to react and prepare to answer questions that you think they might ask you.

Be clear about who they can and cannot share information with about your HIV status with. You don't want to lose control over who knows that you have HIV.

Telling somebody that you have HIV might tap into their prejudices about sexuality, illness, disability, race or HIV itself. Think about how you will react if this happens.

It can be very difficult if the person you tell is very upset or doesn't understand. You might feel like the one offering support. In addition, it's possible that a person may feel under pressure to offer you support and may not know be able to, or know how to.

Telling your partner

If you have spent time discussing having an HIV test with your partner, then you may have a good idea of what their reaction might be. If you didn't discuss having an HIV test with your partner, then think about the practicalities of telling your partner and what their reaction might be. It could be that your HIV status could have health implications for your partner. Telling your partner you have HIV could also put stress on your relationship.

Telling sexual partners

See the section on disclosing your HIV status to sexual partners in the chapter *HIV and the law*.

Telling ex-partners

It can be very difficult telling ex-partners and past sexual contacts that you have HIV. Whether or not you can, or even need to, tell them can depend on a number of factors, such as what your relationship was like with them, the kind of sex you had, whether you think they would want to know and whether you want them to know.

Staff at your HIV clinic can contact your ex-partners and sexual contacts without giving any of your details away.

Family

You may immediately want to tell your family that you have HIV. However, many people find this very difficult. Breaking the news to your family can be distressing for both you and them. There's no right or wrong time to tell your parents, brothers, sisters that you have HIV. Some people tell them immediately, others after years, and some people never tell their family. You know best what and/or when they would like to know, and how and when to tell them.

Friends

It is good to have somebody close to you to confide in when you are upset, confused, angry, or need to talk things through. You may well have a friend who you instinctively know you can trust to tell that you have HIV and look to for support. But you should still take time to think things through. Think about why you want to tell a friend or friends. Consider the likely impact on your friendship of telling them you have HIV. Think about how they may react when you tell them, and about what their reaction would be if they found out from another source after you didn't tell them.

Remember, friends might talk amongst themselves or to other people about your health. It's important to make it clear to them if you want them to keep information about your HIV to themselves.

Work

In most cases, these should be no reason why your employer would need to know that you have HIV. Even if you need to have a lot off time off sick, there is no need for your employer to know that HIV is the cause.

Some employers offer very good support to people with HIV, and the UK Disability Discrimination Act makes it illegal for an HIV-positive person to be discriminated against at work because of their health status.

Healthcare professionals

GPs

Everybody who is HIV-positive should be registered with a GP. In order for your GP to provide the most appropriate care, it is important that they know if you have any serious medical conditions, including HIV, or are taking medicines that a hospital specialist has prescribed to you, such as anti-HIV medication.

GPs are not allowed to refuse to register you because you are HIV-positive, or discriminate against you in any way because you are HIV-positive or because of your sexuality, sex or lifestyle.

A lot of people are concerned that informing their GP that they have HIV could have implications if they apply for a mortgage or life assurance. Your GP records are confidential, but it is true that if you apply for life cover the company will almost certainly ask about your medical history and ask to have access to your GP records. You should be aware, however, that if you fail to tell a life insurance company that you are HIV-positive when you apply for a home loan it could have very serious consequences later.

Your HIV clinic may have a list of recommended GPs in your area.

Dentists

When you register with a dentist, you may be asked to fill out a form describing your medical history. This may ask you if you are HIV-positive and have certain other illnesses such as hepatitis B or C. Alternatively, a dentist may ask you if you're HIV-positive.

According to the professional body for UK dentists, a dentist should not discriminate against you because you disclose your HIV status. Sadly, this has not always been the case. Dentists have sometimes claimed that they have refused treatment in order to protect themselves and their other patients from HIV. This is not acceptable. Standard sterilisation and infection control procedures are sufficient to ensure that no patient poses a risk to dental staff or other patients.

Telling your dentist you have HIV can have benefits. They can know to check for certain gum problems that can occur more often in people with HIV. Also, it is wise to tell your dentist if you are taking any medication prescribed to treat HIV or any other infections, as dentists may need to use drugs that could interact with them.

If you are worried about telling a dentist, then ask your HIV clinic to recommend one. They may even have a specialist HIV dentist. Your dental records are confidential.

Pharmacists

A pharmacist may ask you what medicines you are taking when they dispense a prescription or when you buy over-the-counter medication. Some over-the-counter medicines (medicines available without a doctor's prescription), for example hay fever tablets, can interact dangerously with certain anti-HIV drugs. It can be especially hard to maintain your confidentiality at a High Street pharmacy counter, so if you do need over-the-counter medicines on a regular basis, it might be wise to discuss this with your HIV doctor or specialist HIV pharmacist.

Complementary health practitioners

Many people with HIV use complementary therapists, such as acupuncturists. If you do, you may wish to disclose your health status to them. It should not make a difference to the kind of therapy they offer you.

However, complementary practitioners are not as well regulated as medical professionals. You may wish to check confidentiality policies before disclosing any health details.

If you are advised to take any complementary or alternative therapy, check with your doctor or HIV pharmacist that it is safe. Some alternative medicines, such as the herbal anti-depressant St John's wort, can stop some anti-HIV drugs working properly. Even if you tell a complementary practitioner that you are taking anti-HIV drugs, it is not certain that they will know of any possible dangerous interactions.

Children

Children can be very perceptive and might be worrying if their parent or guardian is ill. They need clear and appropriate information to help them to understand the situation.

You may find that even very young children will want to know why their parent has to go to the doctor a lot or is constantly unwell. It could be useful to talk about "goodies" or "baddies" in the blood, or bugs, which may enable you to talk about illness without actually mentioning HIV. In this way, you can begin to foster an understanding of health and illness which you can build upon, adding more details as the child gets older.

Further reading

NAM factsheet, *Disclosing your HIV status to healthcare workers*.

Do I need to tell anyone about being HIV-positive?, leaflet produced by the Terrence Higgins Trust.

Grateful? I don't think so, by Susan

"You must be so grateful that your partner agreed to stay with you despite the fact that you have, you know, AIDS," said a particularly vacuous journalist to me, during an interview for a women's magazine. "Actually, no," I replied, "He's grateful that I stay with him, because I'm so great in bed." Strangely, she chose to ignore my comment and continued to portray me as a vapid pathetic creature, ashamed of my status and gushing with gratitude that someone would deign to go out with diseased old me. No mention of the fact that I have a remarkable capacity to suppress my gag reflex.

It saddens me when I read about people living with HIV who feel that they have to hang up their shagging shoes and turn to a life of laborious abstinence. Should an HIV-positive diagnosis correlate with an abandoned libido? Well, I must confess that I did have a temporary loss of libido when I was first diagnosed. Being told that I only had four years to live didn't make me feel particularly horny. Perhaps feeling that sex was the cause of my being HIV-positive, coupled with my Catholic conscience issues, put me off the dirty deed for a while.

At the time, I was in a relationship with a particularly vile American. He suggested that no one would want to be with me now, as I was HIV-positive. My self-esteem was so suppressed that I actually believed him. After we split up, I felt that my life would comprise of eating microwave meals for one and masturbation (surprisingly pleasurable if undertaken simultaneously). It took a year of making my eyesight considerably worse (only kidding), before I abandoned that notion.

I met my current partner at a conference and was immediately blinded with lust. I initially believed that our relationship would simply be a short-term sex thing, so didn't feel that it was necessary to disclose my status – we always had protected sex. A month later, I found myself in the heinous position of falling in love. I vacillated with the idea of dumping him, rather than face being rejected when I told him about my positive status. Finally I chose to tell him, classily, in a McDonald's car park (the rationale being that, if he rejected me, I'd have the compensation of a Big Mac Meal).

I began in a somewhat cowardly way, by saying "I have something to tell you about me, that's quite bad", and proceeded to let him guess. His first guess, rather alarmingly, was that I used to be a man – but he finally got there. Instead of rushing off to scrub himself in bleach, he professed his love, and three years later we're still together.

I do hope we'll stay together long-term, but if we don't, I don't think I'll be booking myself into the nearest nunnery quite yet. My self-esteem has rebounded to its previous monstrous proportions – to the extent that I believe most men would be lucky to have me, regardless of my HIV-positive status. Pass me a banana and I'll show you one of the reasons why...

Getting HIV treatment and care

Introduction

In the UK, nearly all HIV treatment and care is provided by specialist hospital clinics. Because HIV has mainly (but not exclusively) been spread through sex in this country, HIV healthcare services in the UK developed through, and are often provided by, genitourinary medicine (GUM) and sexual health clinics. In some parts of the UK, infectious disease or immunology departments developed into specialist HIV clinics. HIV clinics may also be provided through haematology units for people with haemophilia, drug dependency units for injecting drug users, and specialist children's hospitals.

Many HIV treatment centres are in London. This is because the majority of people with HIV live in London. However, there are hospitals offering HIV treatment and care in all the major cities in the UK.

HIV clinics

HIV care is provided through outpatient clinics. This means that you do not receive your treatment whilst staying in hospital, but visit a specialist doctor at regular intervals who will monitor your health, prescribe treatments and, if you need to, refer you to see other specialists.

Many HIV clinics are attached to a GUM clinic, and there's a good chance that you will be receiving your HIV care from the

HIV clinic associated with the GUM clinic where you were diagnosed with HIV.

Unlike any other specialism within the NHS, GUM and HIV clinics operate an open access policy. You don't need your family doctor to refer you. All you have to do is phone up and make an appointment. You can choose which HIV treatment centre you receive your care from. You do not have to attend the clinic at the hospital you were diagnosed at. If you wish, you can use the HIV treatment centre in a different city. If you decide to change clinics, it's very important to ensure that your medical notes are forwarded from your old clinic to your new one.

If you are entitled to free NHS care, then all the treatment you receive from your HIV clinic will be free. Even if you normally have to pay for prescriptions, nearly all medicines prescribed by a specialist HIV doctor will be free.

It's likely that as well as regular appointments with a doctor who specialises in the treatment of HIV, your clinic will have other specialist services available to you. There will almost certainly be a specialist HIV pharmacist. There's also a good chance that there might be nurse-led clinics looking after sexual health, or supporting adherence to drug regimens. The very large HIV clinics may also have specialist HIV mental health teams, and access to dentists.

An emergency walk-in doctor service is provided by some clinics during normal working hours. This is intended for problems requiring urgent medical attention.

Opening times vary between clinics. You can expect the very large clinics to be open and to offer appointments with doctors and other health professionals every working day. By contrast, smaller clinics might only be open a few mornings or afternoons a week.

All clinics will have arrangements for providing emergency care. The large HIV clinics will have an HIV doctor who is on call 24 hours a day for an emergency, while at smaller hospitals emergency cover might be provided by a general medicine doctor.

The factors influencing choice of clinic differ from person to person. Some might prefer to attend a clinic that is large, with a reputation for expertise. Others opt to attend smaller clinics that are more accessible and convenient.

Whichever clinic you attend, it's very important that you receive appropriate treatment and care that you are comfortable with. If you are not satisfied with the level of service you are receiving, then complain to the clinic management. Set out clearly what you are unhappy about. An advocacy organisation might be able to help. Try not to get angry, and don't get abusive. The chances are that your complaint will be settled satisfactorily. If your complaint isn't settled to your satisfaction, then remember you can change to a different clinic.

Your HIV clinic will also have facilities to treat inpatients (treatment whilst staying in hospital). Large clinics are likely to have a dedicated HIV ward with doctors and nurses who only treat HIV-positive patients. If you attend a smaller clinic, then inpatient care is likely to be provided on a general medical or infectious diseases ward.

Staff on specialist inpatient wards may well have more insight into the medical and psychological issues faced by people with HIV, and will have more skill at recognising and treating both the common and uncommon illnesses and complications seen in people with HIV. Other staff at hospitals with a large HIV clinic, such as pharmacists, dieticians, radiologists and physiotherapists will also have extensive experience of treating HIV-positive patients.

It's worth bearing in mind that the large HIV clinics, which have lots of patients and more expertise, have better survival and outcome rates for their patients. To put it simply: if you go to a large clinic with experienced staff, you improve your chances of living a longer, healthier life.

If you are admitted to hospital for a reason unconnected to HIV, it's very important to let the doctors and nurses looking after you know that you are HIV-positive, to ensure that you receive the right treatment.

You and your doctor

The relationship you forge with your specialist HIV doctor is one of the most important you will have after your diagnosis.

Certain doctors may attract certain kinds of patients: some doctors will advocate aggressive therapy, whilst others will be more receptive should you wish to hold off treatment or use a range of complementary approaches in addition to conventional HIV care.

It's important that you find the right kind of doctor for you. Friends who are HIV-positive may be able to recommend a suitable doctor, but building up a relationship will take time. You may not develop a rapport with the first doctor you meet. Establishing a trusting relationship with your doctor is essential if you are to feel empowered and in control of your use of treatments.

Your doctor should have good interpersonal skills. The level of knowledge of your clinician is clearly important too. An effective doctor should take the trouble to explain things to you, be sensitive to personal issues raised by you, be a good listener and be able to provide you with a range of opinions.

All patients need their doctors to be open, frank and communicative – as well as honest when he or she does not know the answer to your questions.

You will need to be involved in your own care. Exactly what this means depends upon the type of person you are. Some people will want to take a more active role in their health care. They may have clear ideas about what kind of treatments they do or do not want to use. Others will be more inclined to look to their doctor for guidance.

Being prepared for your consultations is a joint responsibility. Keep asking questions until you understand. If you are likely to forget what your doctor tells you during the consultation, make notes. If you are likely to forget which questions you would like to ask, then write a letter to your doctor containing the questions you want to ask, and send it in advance of your appointment. It's also worth remembering that if you attend your clinic without an appointment, your regular doctor may not be available.

During the course of your relationship with your doctor, it's likely there will occasionally be issues upon which you do not agree. It's important that you learn how to manage these situations. If you become unhappy over a disagreement with your doctor, you may choose to invite a patient advocate to help you communicate your feelings.

It is important to be honest with your doctor about any risks you may be taking, or sexual practices, alcohol or drug use that may affect your long-term health. Knowing the facts helps your doctor to consider appropriate care and treatment for you. If, however, you feel unable to confide in your doctor about certain issues, there may be other staff in the department who you could talk to more easily.

Maintaining contact with the same doctor can be extremely difficult, as they are usually very busy, and staff change from time to time. Remember though, their time is no more valuable than your own. If getting access to your doctor is difficult, discuss ways of improving the situation. Would a short phone call or e-mail enquiry be acceptable? You will need to be organised to get the most from your doctor's time. Learning about the roles of other staff at your treatment centre will also help you avoid using your doctor's time when another member of staff would be able to help, and can provide you with additional sources of support. For some non-HIV-related medical problems, it might be more appropriate to see a GP.

GPs

Even though you receive your HIV care from a specialist HIV clinic, it is still important to have a GP. Firstly, many GPs offer services which are not available at your HIV clinic, but which you may need from time to time, such as health visiting for women who have recently had a baby; district nurses, if you need nursing support at home; mental health nursing; physiotherapy and chiropody.

GPs are able to provide prescriptions for non-HIV medicines which your clinic may be unable to supply for more than a couple of weeks. Also, GPs are the only doctors who can make home visits if you are too ill to attend your HIV clinic or your GP's surgery. If you are unwell outside normal working hours, or at the weekend or bank holidays, all GPs have an emergency service through which a nurse or doctor will offer advice and, if necessary, visit you at home. If the problem is very serious and requires hospital care, they can arrange for your admission into hospital and will normally be willing to speak to the on-call HIV doctor at your clinic to arrange specialist HIV care if appropriate.

To get access to a GP you must be registered as their patient. You can only be registered with one GP and you must live within the area the GP practices in. When you register you will be asked to give your name and address, your NHS number and details of your last GP. Don't worry if you can't find your NHS number, you can still register without it. A few weeks after you register with a GP you will receive a card confirming your registration, which will have your NHS number on it.

Most HIV clinics keep a list of GPs, and may be able to recommend a GP with experience of caring for people with HIV. However, GPs often find that they cannot accept any more patients, as they already have on their register the maximum number of people to whom they can offer services. You can also contact NHS Direct on 0845 4647 for details of all GP practices in your area. If you still have problems finding a GP who is able to register you, then contact your local Community Health

Council. GPs cannot refuse to register you because you have HIV or any other medical condition, or because of your race, colour or sexuality. It's also worth remembering that many GPs, particularly those with practices outside cities and big towns, may have a very limited knowledge of HIV and will have seen very few HIV-positive patients.

If you need a GP when you are away from home, then you can register as a 'temporary resident' if you will be within their practice area for 14 days or less.

If you are entitled to free NHS treatment, then all NHS services provided by your GP will be free. GPs are not obliged to provide free NHS treatment to people who are visiting the UK from abroad or who do not have the legal right to stay in the UK. GPs also provide some other services for a fee, such as signing passport applications.

Most GPs have an appointment system, and sometimes these become booked up for weeks in advance. Emergency appointments will usually be available for people who need to be seen quickly. These are normally available the same day, but on a 'first come, first served' basis.

If you don't disclose your HIV status to your GP, you must be aware that this may prevent you from receiving the best care. For example, if you are taking HIV drugs, it's important to consider potentially harmful interactions with other medications. Your GP medical records are confidential, and nobody can see them without your consent. If you are concerned about disclosing your status, explore whether staff at your HIV treatment centre, or an advocate, could help you assess your GP's practice around disclosure beforehand.

Dentists

There have been cases where people with HIV have been refused treatment by a dentist. Dentists in the UK have been told by their governing body that they cannot refuse to treat somebody just because they are HIV-positive. General hygiene precautions are enough to prevent the transmission of HIV during dental treatment.

As with all healthcare workers, it's a good idea to let them know if you have any serious medical conditions or are taking any medication. This will help them ensure that you receive the most appropriate treatment. It is wrong for dentists or any other health professional to discriminate against you because of your health status, race, or sexuality.

Not all dentists offer NHS care, and in some parts of the UK there are long waiting lists to register with NHS dentists.

Your HIV clinic might be able to help you find an NHS dentist, or a dentist that is particularly skilled or interested in treating people with HIV. Some of the large HIV clinics even have their own dental clinics.

Regular visits to the dentist are recommended for people with HIV. Not only will this ensure that your general dental health is being looked after, but it will also allow dentists to look for gum and mouth disorders, such as oral thrush and badly bleeding gums, which can occur more frequently in people with HIV.

NHS care and non-UK nationals

There is no general right to come to the UK in order to obtain free treatment from the UK's National Health Service (NHS). Nationals of the member states of the European Economic Area (EEA), or their family members, and refugees and stateless persons living within the EEA, have the right to NHS treatment without charge where the need arises during their stay. EEA nationals who wish to enter the UK for treatment (or who are referred to the UK for treatment) should obtain prior authorisation from their national social security institution, which in principle bears the cost, and obtain form E112 before travelling. (The EEA member states are: Austria, Belgium, Denmark, Finland, France, Germany, Greece, Iceland, Ireland, Italy, Liechtenstein, Luxembourg, Netherlands, Norway, Portugal, Spain, and Sweden).

Most NHS treatment is not automatically free of charge to other people from abroad. Access to the NHS depends on a combination of one or more of: immigration status; length of residence; nature of the treatment required; and whether the need for it arose during the visit.

However, certain NHS treatment is free to anyone at all. This includes testing and counselling for HIV or sexually transmitted infections at a genitourinary clinic (but not any subsequent treatment for HIV), family planning services, treatment for mental disorders, hospital accident and emergency treatment (but not in-patient care) and treatment for notifiable diseases and other conditions to which public health laws apply (not including HIV and AIDS).

In addition, certain categories of people are exempt from any NHS charges. The main categories are: anyone in employment in the UK; anyone taking up permanent residence in the UK; anyone who has resided in the UK for twelve months; refugees and asylum seekers; prisoners and immigration detainees; full-time students; those covered by a reciprocal agreement with a country listed in schedule 2 (see below).

Other categories of people are exempt from charges for treatment, if the need for it arose during a visit to the UK. This provision is intended to exclude travel to the UK specifically for treatment on the NHS of a pre-existing condition. This group consists mainly of European Union citizens and their dependants, and residents from the countries listed in schedule 2.

Schedule 2 countries are: Anguilla, Australia, Barbados, British Virgin Islands, Bulgaria, Channel Islands, Czech Republic, Falkland Islands, Gibraltar, Hungary, Isle of Man, Malta, Montserrat, New Zealand, Poland, Romania, Russia and former USSR states (excluding Latvia, Lithuania and Estonia), Slovak Republic, St Helena, Turks and Caicos Islands, and states of the former Yugoslavia (Serbia, Montenegro, Croatia, Bosnia, Slovenia, Macedonia).

The NHS regulations refer only to hospital treatment, but GPs, dentists and opticians are advised to apply corresponding criteria in deciding whether or not to accept patients for treatment under the NHS.

Immigration is a complex and specialist topic, and the the law can change quickly. It is essential that anyone seeking information on this subject go to appropriate advice agencies. The following organisations can provide guidance:

• Joint Council for the Welfare of Immigrants, 115 Old St, London EC1V 9JR, 020 251 8706(advice line).

• Refugee Legal Centre, Sussex House, 39-45 Bermondsey Street, London SE1, 020 7780 3220 (advice line), Open for individual advice on Mon, Tue, Wed and Fri 9.30am – 1.00pm and 2pm – 4pm.

• Immigration Law Practitioners Association, Lindsey House, 40-42 Charterhouse Street, London EC1M 6JN, 020 7251 8383.

• THT Advice Centre, contact via THT Direct 0845 1221 200.

• Immigration and Nationality Directorate, www. ind.homeoffice.gov.uk.

• Citizens Advice Bureau, www.citizensadvice.org.uk.

Further reading

NAM factsheets: *GPs and primary care, HIV clinic services, NHS and non-UK nationals,* and *You and your doctor.*

GPs – why bother?

I really didn't see that there was any point having a GP. My regular check-ups at my HIV clinic seemed more than sufficient to take care of not only my HIV-related health problems, but my routine healthcare needs as well.

On top of this, I'd had a bad experience a number of years earlier with a GP who'd said some really anti-gay things to me. I told myself that it would be no great loss if I didn't register with one, even though I was asked who my GP was every time I went to my HIV clinic.

One Saturday morning, however, I awoke with a fever, a temperature of 101 degrees and a cough. As it was the weekend, I knew that my HIV clinic would be closed and that I wouldn't be able to use its walk-in emergency doctor. Nevertheless, I called the hospital and asked to speak to the HIV ward for advice. They told me to call my GP. When I explained I didn't have one, they said that the only way I could get to see a doctor would be to come into Casualty and wait.

I didn't fancy experiencing at first hand the long delays which the media is always reporting and decided that I was well enough to wait until Monday morning. I wasn't. By Monday morning, when I finally saw a doctor, my temperature was temperature was a constant 104 degrees.

After a chest x-ray I was admitted to hospital with PCP, which was successfully treated.

One of the first things I did after coming home was register with a GP. By and large, my fears have proved unfounded. Although my GP is interested in my HIV and its treatment, she leaves it entirely in the hands of the HIV specialists. I've not detected any prejudice. And, the last time I became ill – again at a weekend – it was my GP who, after a home visit, was able to arrange my speedy admission to hospital.

Charlotte's story

Charlotte had arranged to stay with friends in London while she waited for the results of her application for asylum. When she was diagnosed HIV-positive, Charlotte says, "I started crying and I cried for weeks." Her situation worsened when her friends found out about her status. "I told my friends and... oh my God. They began to mistreat me. They didn't want me to touch anything, to use the bathroom or the kitchen and when I went to the toilet, they would flush it about ten times afterwards. They thought they would catch it off me."

Charlotte had become ill, but the treatment came quickly and was effective. In the past few months, her CD4 count has risen to over 50 from just three when she was first diagnosed. Her viral load is now undetectable after peaking at 700,000. "Since I've been on medication I've changed because I feel so well," she explains.

However, Charlotte's physical health has been somewhat jeopardised by the pressures of securing a new life in London. Her friends threw her out, so she went to the social services to enquire about accommodation.

Recent policy changes have meant that all asylum seekers are housed outside of London. A spokesperson from the Refugee Arrivals Project said that: "Although RAP is based in London, the asylum seekers who come to us do not stay long enough for them to access the services available in the area. Clients who are HIV-positive did not receive any special treatment and were dispersed with others." For Charlotte, this would have meant disrupting her treatment, which was just beginning to control the virus. Charlotte's doctor stepped in and appealed on her behalf, and since then Charlotte has been able to stay in London.

Just before Christmas, Charlotte was allocated a room in a Bed and Breakfast in west London. The one meal provided every day coincides with the time she has to take her medication, on an empty stomach. "By the time I can eat, the dining room is closed and I have nowhere to prepare food. So sometimes I take my medication, but then don't eat. Sometimes I have to miss taking my medication totally."

Receiving £36 in food vouchers per week, and having nowhere to prepare fresh food, means that Charlotte must often rely on convenience food, which is also adding to any problems she may experience with her health. "My doctor told me my cholesterol is too high," she says.

Without access to a fridge, Charlotte says that she is 'lucky' that it is so cold outside, because she can keep her medications cool. Every morning she gets up very early, before they clean the streets, to retrieve her stash of medications from the plants outside where she hides them.

Nic Alderson, who works for the Inter Agency Co-ordination Team that oversees six refugee projects across the UK, explains the problem of accommodating asylum seekers: "It was expected that asylum seekers would stay seven days in emergency accommodation, but that has become a bit of an nonsense. It now averages between 20 and 50 days. Emergency accommodation in London is full. Combine this with people staying longer, and there just isn't enough support for people."

Despite her problems, Charlotte says she is 'happy' that she came to London, because she is not ill anymore. For the future, she wants "a proper place to live – with HIV you need privacy. If I could work, I would rent a house for myself and be independent. But I can't work until my application for asylum has been considered – they won't give me a permit."

I feel frustrated for Charlotte, but I don't think Charlotte sees it that way: "Right now I'm doing well," she tells me, "I don't fall sick. I meet other women at Positively Women. And I don't cry anymore."

This testimony first appeared on the website of Positively Women, www.positivelywomen.org.uk. Thanks to both the writer and Positively Women for giving permission to reprint it here.

Key tests to monitor HIV – CD4 and viral load

Why monitor?

There are two key tests that doctors use to assess how HIV is affecting your body.

The CD4 cell count is a guide to how strong your immune system is. The viral load test measures the amount of HIV in your blood.

Regular monitoring of CD4 cell count and HIV viral load provide a good indication of the effects of HIV on your body. Doctors can interpret your test results in the context of what they know about the course of HIV disease progression.

For example, your risk of developing opportunistic infections is directly related to your CD4 cell count. The level of your viral load predicts how rapidly your CD4 cell count is likely to fall. Looked at together, these two results can be used to predict your risk of developing AIDS in the next few years. For example, if your HIV viral load is above 55,000 and your CD4 cell count below 200, then there's an 85% chance that you'll develop AIDS in the next three years. This is illustrated in the table on the next page.

Results from your CD4 cell count and viral load tests can help you and your doctor make decisions about when to take HIV treatments, or therapy to help prevent you from developing opportunistic infections.

There are different testing methods used to measure viral load. When your viral load is first tested, ask the doctor which method was being used. Was it:

- Roche Amplicor Ultrasensitive HIV-1 monitor

or

- Chiron Quantiplex b-DNA version 3.0.

Predicting progression
% of people who develop AIDS within 3 years (assuming no treatment)

Viral load		CD4				
Roche test	Chiron test	below 200	201-350	351-500	501-750	above 750
below 1,500	below 500	**	**	**	3.7	0
1,500-7,000	500-3,000	**	**	2.0	2.0	2.0
7,000-20,000	3,000-10,000	**	8.1	8.1	8.1	3.2
20,000-55,000	10,000-30,000	40.1	40.1	16.1	16.1	9.5
above 55,000	above 30,000	85.5	64.4	42.9	32.6	32.6

** indicates lack of data

CD4 cell counts

What CD4 cells do
CD4 cells, sometimes also called T-cells, or T-helper cells, are white blood cells which organise the immune system's response to bacterial, fungal and viral infections.

CD4 cell counts in people without HIV
A normal CD4 cell count in an HIV-negative man is between 400 and 1600 per cubic millimetre of blood. CD4 cell counts in HIV-negative women tend to be a little higher, between 500 – 1600.

Even if you don't have HIV, many factors can affect your CD4 cell count. For example it's known that:

- Women have higher CD4 cell counts than men (by about 100).

- Women's CD4 cell counts go up and down during the menstrual cycle.

- Oral contraceptives can lower a woman's CD4 cell count.

- Smokers tend to have higher CD4 cell counts (by about 140).

- CD4 cell counts fall after rest – by as much as 40%.

- A good night's sleep can mean that you have a lower CD4 cell count the following morning, but a higher CD4 cell count the next afternoon.

None of these factors seems to make any difference to how able your immune system is to fight infections.

Only a small portion of your body's CD4 cells are in the blood. The rest are in the lymph nodes and tissue, and the fluctuations noted above might be due to the movement of CD4 cells between blood and tissue.

CD4 cell counts in people with HIV

Soon after infection with HIV, your CD4 cell count probably dropped sharply, before stabilising at around 500 – 600. It seems that people who experience a greater initial drop in CD4 cell count and a lower stabilisation in their CD4 cell count may be at risk of faster disease progression. Even while you are well and have no obvious symptoms of HIV, millions of CD4 cells are infected by HIV and lost every day, and millions more are produced to replace them.

It's estimated, however, that without treatment, an HIV-positive person's CD4 cell count drops by about 45 cells every six months, with greater falls experienced by people with higher CD4 cell counts.

A CD4 cell count between 200 and 500 indicates that some damage to your immune system has occurred.

Steeper falls in CD4 cell counts are experienced in the year before AIDS develops, which is why you are recommended to have your CD4 cell count regularly monitored once it goes below 350.

Looking at your CD4 cell count can also provide a guide for decisions about your need to take medicines to prevent some AIDS-defining illnesses. For example, if your CD4 cell count is below 200, you are recommended to take antibiotics to prevent you getting PCP pneumonia.

Your CD4 cell count can naturally fluctuate, so don't put too much emphasis on a single test result. Rather, look at the trend in a number of recent CD4 cell counts.

If your CD4 cell count is high, you have no symptoms, and are not taking anti-HIV medication, then it probably only needs monitoring every few months or so.

However, if it's falling rapidly, you are unwell, are taking part in a clinical trial, or are taking anti-HIV drugs, then it should be monitored more often.

CD4 cell percentages

Sometimes, as well as counting the number of CD4 cells, doctors will also assess what percentage of all your white blood cells are CD4 cells. This is called the CD4 cell percentage. A normal result in a person with an intact immune system is about 40%, and a CD4 cell percentage below 20% indicates the same risk of becoming ill with an AIDS-defining illness as a CD4 cell count of about 200.

CD4 cell counts and HIV treatment

Your CD4 cell count can be used to help decide when you need to start anti-HIV treatment, and as an indication of how successful these treatments are.

Once your CD4 cell falls to about 350, your doctor should start talking to you about whether you need to start taking anti-HIV treatments.

If your CD4 cell count falls to between 200 and 250 cells, you are recommended to start anti-HIV treatment. A CD4 cell count of this level indicates that you are at a real risk of becoming ill with an AIDS-defining illness.

It also seems that if you wait until your CD4 cell count falls to below 200, you are less likely to respond well to anti-HIV treatment. However, there doesn't seem to be any health benefit from starting HIV treatment if your CD4 cell count is above 350.

Once you start anti-HIV treatment, your CD4 cell count should start to slowly increase. If you experience a fall in your CD4 cell count over a number of tests, this should alert your doctor that there's something wrong with your HIV treatments.

Viral load

What is viral load?

Viral load is the amount of HIV in the blood.

The more HIV you have in your blood, the faster your CD4 cell count will fall, and the greater your risk of developing symptoms of HIV infection or AIDS-defining illnesses.

People taking anti-HIV drugs normally see an increase in their CD4 cell count as viral load falls. If you're taking treatment, monitoring your viral load gives an indication of how well your treatments are working.

What is the viral load test?

Viral load tests estimate the number of HIV particles circulating in the liquid, or plasma, part of the blood. They do this by looking for HIV's genes, which are called HIV RNA.

The result of a viral load test is described as the number of copies of HIV RNA per millilitre. For example, a viral load of two hundred would be written as 200 copies/ml. But your doctor is likely to describe your viral load using just the number.

There are several different viral load tests, or assays, in use at the moment. These tests use different techniques to measure the number of HIV particles, but the tests are equally reliable at showing whether your viral load is low, medium, or high. The PCR (polymerase chain reaction) assay is the one most commonly used in the UK.

Viral load tests used in this country are equally accurate at measuring types of HIV (called subtypes) found in other parts of the world, for example Africa and Asia.

It's now usual to use what are called ultra-sensitive viral load tests. These are able to detect viral load as low as 50 copies/ml. If your viral load is below 50 copies/ml, it is said to be 'undetectable' and, for most people, getting an undetectable viral load is one of the key goals of anti-HIV treatment. This is considered in a lot more detail in the chapter *Anti-HIV treatment.*

Understanding your viral load results

A viral load above 100,000 copies/ml is considered high, and one below 10,000 copies/ml is considered low.

But your viral load can seem to fluctuate quite widely from one test to another if you are not on treatment, even though this has no implications for your health.

Indeed, doctors have looked at viral load changes in people not on anti-HIV treatment and have found that two separate tests on the same sample of blood can give widely different results. So you shouldn't get too worried if your viral load increases from 5,000 copies/ml to 15,000 copies/ml when you're not on treatment. Even an increase from 50,000 copies/ml to 100,000 copies/ml isn't necessarily that important if you're not on treatment. Although it appears that your viral load might have doubled, it's within the margin of error for the test.

Rather than attaching too much importance to a single viral load test result, look at the trend in your viral load over time. The time of day your blood sample is taken could influence your viral load, and your viral load might temporarily increase if you're unwell with an infection before falling back again. Similarly, some vaccinations can cause a temporary variation in your viral load.

You should, however, be concerned if your viral load results over several months show an upward trend, or if the increase is greater than threefold. For example, an increase from 5,000 to 15,000 isn't significant, but an increase from 5,000 to 25,000 is.

Undetectable viral load

All viral load tests have a cut-off point below which they cannot reliably detect HIV. This is called the limit of detection, and the tests used in the UK have a lower limit of detection of 50 copies/ml. If your viral load is below 50 it is said to be undetectable.

But just because the level of HIV is too low to be measured doesn't mean that HIV has disappeared from your blood. It might still be present in the blood, but in amounts too low to be measured. As viral load tests only measure levels of HIV in the blood, the viral load in other parts of your body, for example your lymph nodes or sexual fluids, might be detectable.

Why it's good to have an undetectable viral load

Having an undetectable viral load is desirable for two reasons. It means that you are at a very low risk of becoming ill because of HIV, and also that there is a very low risk that you will become resistant to your anti-HIV treatments.

HIV can only become resistant to a drug if it continues to reproduce whilst you are taking that drug. If the reproduction of HIV is kept at very low levels, the appearance of drug resistance should be delayed, perhaps indefinitely. This means that your anti-HIV drugs go on working.

Because of this, HIV doctors now stress that an aim of anti-HIV treatment should be to get HIV viral load down to undetectable levels as soon as possible, ideally within 24 weeks of starting HIV treatment.

Some people take three to six months to reach this point, others go below detection within four to twelve weeks, and others may never reach this goal.

For a discussion on whether people who have an undetectable viral load are infectious, see the section *Sex and HIV*

Viral load blips

If your viral load is undetectable, there's a good chance that your viral load might occasionally increase above 50 copies/ml to 100 or 200 copies/ml in a single test before falling back to being undetectable. These are called viral load blips and they do not indicate that your anti-HIV treatment is failing. Indeed, most blips seem to be due to testing errors at the laboratory.

Viral load in women

Women seem to have lower viral loads than men with the same CD4 cell counts. This doesn't have any effect on the rate of HIV disease progression and the reasons for it aren't properly understood. It's been suggested that women might have lower viral loads due to a superior immune response to infections; or that viral production is naturally lower in women.

Looking at CD4 and viral load together

If you're not currently taking anti-HIV treatment

If you're not currently taking anti-HIV threatment, your viral load and CD4 cell count can help predict your risk of becoming ill because of HIV in the future.

Among people with the same CD4 cell counts, research has shown that those with a higher viral load tend to develop symptoms more quickly than those with a lower viral load.

In addition, among people with the same viral load, those with lower CD4 cell counts tend to become ill more quickly.

As the table in the section 'Why monitor?' earlier in this chapter shows, looked at together, your CD4 cell count and viral load provide an indication of your risk of developing AIDS in the short to medium term.

For example, if you look at the column for people with a CD4 cell count between 351 and 500 you can see that there is a big variation in the risk of disease progression, depending on the level of viral load.

Deciding when to start treatment

Your viral load and CD4 cell count can help you decide if you need to start taking anti-HIV treatment.

At the moment, doctors put more emphasis on the level of your CD4 cell count, and it is recommended that you start treatment before your CD4 cell count falls below 200. This is because your risk of death is greater if you start treatment when your CD4 cell count is below 200.

At higher CD4 cell counts, the picture is much less clear, and your decision will depend on a combination of the level of your viral load, the speed at which your CD4 cell count is falling, any symptoms you may have, and your wishes.

The question of when to start HIV treatment is looked at in a lot more detail in the chapter *Anti-HIV treatment*.

Monitoring the effectiveness of treatment

Effective anti-HIV treatment results in a fall in your viral load. Within about four weeks of starting HIV treatment, your doctor should test your viral load to see how much it has fallen.

The aim of treatment in people who have never taken anti-HIV drugs before is to get viral load to undetectable levels within 24 weeks.

As your viral load falls, your CD4 cell count should begin to slowly increase.

Frequency of testing

If you're not on treatment

Even if your CD4 cell count is above 500, it's a good idea to go to your HIV clinic every three to six months for a CD4 cell count and viral load test. Make sure you go back promptly for your results.

If your CD4 cell count is between 200 and 350, you'll need to go to your clinic every couple of months, or even monthly, to have your CD4 cell count and viral load checked.

If you're about to start treatment

You should be given a 'baseline' CD4 cell count and two viral load measurements close together shortly before starting treatment. You and your doctors will then be able to assess how effective your treatment has been, by looking at how much your viral load has fallen and your CD4 cell count has risen.

If you're on treatment

You should have your viral load and CD4 cell count measured a month after starting treatment and then about three months after that.

Subsequent CD4 cell counts and viral load tests should be carried out every ten to twelve weeks. Additional tests might be needed if you feel unwell or develop symptoms.

If your viral load increases whilst you are on treatment, you should have a further test within a week or two to confirm this, and your CD4 cell count should be monitored at the same time to see if there's been a fall.

Other tests

As well as monitoring your CD4 cell count and viral load, it's highly likely that you'll have other blood tests as well. Details of the some of the tests you can expect to have are provided below.

Blood counts

Doctors conduct blood counts to see if you are at risk of anaemia (a shortage of red blood cells).

Anaemia can be caused as a result of HIV disease itself. The nucleoside analogue (NRTI) AZT (zidovudine, *Retrovir*) can cause anaemia. The protease inhibitor indinavir (*Crixivan*) has been linked to a small number of cases of anaemia.

Liver function tests

It's very likely that you'll have regular blood tests to monitor the function of your liver.

The non nucleoside analogue nevirapine (*Viramune*) can be toxic to the liver, as can protease inhibitors. Medicines used to treat other infections that people with HIV are vulnerable to can also cause liver problems.

Your doctor is likely to monitor your liver particularly closely if you are also infected with hepatitis B virus or hepatitis C virus (serious viruses which affect the liver).

Many people with HIV only discovered that they were infected with either (or both) hepatitis B or C because they had an abnormal liver function test result and were tested for the presence of these viruses.

Liver function tests look for levels of proteins in the blood, including serum albumin and bilirubin. Other liver function tests include asessing alanine aminotransferase (ALT) and aspartate aminotransferase (AST).

Metabolic tests

Levels of cholesterol (fats) in the blood can be disturbed by anti-HIV drugs, particularly protease inhibitors. Triglycerides, blood sugars, and glucose can also be affected by HIV drugs. You are likely to have tests to monitor the level of your cholesterol, triglycerides and glucose just before you start anti-HIV drugs and then again every time you attend the clinic thereafter.

Liver function tests can give an indication if you have the rare but very serious side-effect lactic acidosis. This can be caused by some drugs in the NRTI class.

Blood samples may also be measured to check levels of the enzyme amylase. Abnormal levels of amylase can be a warning sign that you are at risk of the very serious side-effect pancreatitis. This can be caused by some NRTI drugs.

Kidney function test

Tests will also be conducted to see how well your kidneys are working, particularly if you are taking the protease inhibitor indinavir (*Crixivan*) or the nucleotide analogue tenofovir (*Viread*), as both these drugs are known to cause kidney problems.

Syphilis

If you are sexually active with more than one partner, your clinic may well test you regularly for syphilis. Recent outbreaks of syphilis in several cities in the UK, Europe, and American have been focused on HIV-positive gay men.

Further reading

NAM factsheet, *CD4 T-cell counts, Immune system cells* and *Viral load.*

CD4 and viral load, booklet produced by NAM.

'Viral load, CD4 cell counts and other tests' in NAM's *HIV and AIDS Treatments Directory.*

Anti-HIV treatment

Treatment, not a cure

There is no cure for HIV. However, when taken properly, combinations of different antiretroviral drugs can reduce the amount of HIV in the blood to levels so low that they cannot be detected using the tests that we currently have.

Reducing the amount of HIV, or HIV viral load, has been shown to reduce the risk of becoming ill or dying because of HIV. So, reducing HIV viral load, and keeping it low, is the aim of anti-HIV treatment.

In the UK and the US, the aim of HIV treatment is to get and maintain an undetectable viral load – i.e. a viral load below 50, the cut-off point for the ultrasensitive tests in routine use.

As your HIV viral load goes down, your immune system will start to recover. This should be indicated by an increase in your CD4 cell count, and there's also a good chance that you'll notice an improvement in your health at the same time, if you have been ill due to HIV.

If you have taken lots of HIV drugs, and still have a detectable viral load, then the aim of your treatment might be to boost your CD4 cell count to protect you from infections rather than to achieve an undetectable viral load.

Some researchers have looked at whether treatment with anti-HIV drugs can eliminate, or eradicate, HIV from the body. It was thought by some doctors that treatment during the very early stages of HIV might offer the best chance of achieving this. But even though treatment with powerful combinations of anti-HIV drugs can be successful at getting viral load down to very low levels, HIV will still infect cells and reproduce itself at those very low levels. Anti-HIV drugs can't kill these cells. This means that, with the currently available drugs, eradication of HIV is not possible.

Even when HIV is being suppressed to undetectable low levels, the remaining virus could rebound to high levels if you stop taking your anti-HIV drugs. What's more, anti-HIV drugs are less good at controlling HIV replication in the brain.

When to start treatment

It's not known for certain what is the best time to start treatment with anti-HIV drugs. This means you need to weigh up with your doctor, on an individual basis, the likely benefits and risks of starting treatment now as opposed to waiting until later.

However, it's currently recommended in UK HIV treatment guidelines that you start anti-HIV treatments immediately if you are ill because of HIV, or have an AIDS-defining illness. It's also recommended that you start treatment if your CD4 cell count is near or below 200, the level at which you become vulnerable to serious AIDS-defining illnesses, or is falling very rapidly.

UK treatment guidelines also make other recommendations about whether you should take HIV treatments, depending on the length of time you have been infected with HIV, the level of your CD4 cell count and the amount of HIV in your blood – your viral load.

Recently infected with HIV?

The six months after you are infected by HIV is called primary HIV infection. There is no proof that taking treatment at this time will mean that you live a longer, healthier life. Some doctors believe, however, that treatment at this time may offer a unique chance to control HIV which may be lost later, as your immune system sustains ongoing damage due to HIV, and becomes less able to attack HIV. Whatever your CD4 cell count, if you are considering treatment soon after infection, you should start as soon as possible, and certainly within six months of infection with HIV. Clinical trials are underway to assess the effectiveness of taking anti-HIV treatment at this stage and you might wish to consider joining one.

The potential benefits of taking treatment at this time need to be weighed up against the risk of side-effects. Treatments may reduce your quality of life at a time when HIV would not have. There is also a possibility that if your treatments don't work effectively against HIV, drug resistance could develop, and you would have fewer drug options if you became ill because of HIV.

A very small number of people become really quite ill during primary infection with HIV, and might even need to be admitted to hospital. Taking anti-HIV treatment at this stage may be particularly beneficial in these circumstances. But it's not clear how long you'll need to take treatment for − current practice is to treat for six months to a year − and you might experience symptoms again once you stop your treatment.

Infected with HIV for over six months, but without symptoms?

If your CD4 cell count is above 350, then you are recommended to wait and take treatment later.

However, if your CD4 cell count is between 200 and 350, the picture is much less clear. Large studies of people who have started anti-HIV treatment with different CD4 cell counts suggest that there's no benefit to be had from starting treatment at 350 as opposed to 200.

There are some circumstances when you might want to consider taking treatment if your CD4 cell count is above 200. If your CD4 cell count is falling by more than 80 cells a year then it's likely that your CD4 cell count will fall below 200 in the near future, so starting treatment could be wise. Similarly, you may wish to take treatments now if you have a high viral load, as a high viral load will mean that you lose CD4 cells more rapidly.

Being infected with hepatitis C virus (HCV) is another circumstance in which you may wish to consider starting treatment early. Current treatment guidelines recommend treating your hepatitis C first if your HIV is not making you unwell. There's a lot more information on hepatitis C in the section 'Illnesses in the age of anti-HIV treatment – hepatitis C' in *Symptoms and illnesses*.

Delaying treatment reduces both the impact of long-term side-effects and the risk of developing drug resistance. Treatments in the future might be easier to take, have fewer side-effects, and be more effective against HIV. The best responses to anti-HIV treatment are seen in people who are taking their first combination, so starting too early, or with the wrong combination, could mean that you don't make the most of this best chance.

If your doctor advises you to start treatment but you decide to wait until later, then make sure that you go to your clinic for regular monitoring, at least every two months, and possibly even monthly.

Infected with HIV for over six months, and ill because of HIV?

Regardless of your CD4 cell count, doctors recommend that you should take anti-HIV treatments if you are becoming ill because of HIV.

Similarly, if your CD4 cell count is below 200 you should start anti-HIV treatment immediately.

Starting anti-HIV treatment

Most people who are taking anti-HIV drugs will take a combination, or 'regimen', of three drugs. There are exceptions to this, for example pregnant women (see the chapter *Symptoms and illnesses*), or those who have a very high viral load and need to take more than three drugs to obtain a powerful anti-HIV effect.

Anti-HIV drug classes and names

There are currently 18 drugs licensed for the treatment of HIV, and these drugs are divided into one of four classes depending on how they attack HIV.

Listed below are the classes of drug and the individual drugs within each class. Anti-HIV drugs tend to have more than one name. Listed first is the name the drug is normally called by in this country, then in brackets the generic name for the drug is listed, and finally the drug company's patented tradename for the drug.

Nucleoside analogue reverse transcriptase inhibitors (NRTI, or Nukes for short)

Drugs in this class include AZT (zidovudine, *Retrovir*), ddC (zalcitabine, *Hivid*), ddI (didanosine, *Videx*), 3TC (lamivudine, *Epivir*), d4T (stavudine, *Zerit*), abacavir (*Ziagen*), and FTC (emtricitabine, *Emtriva*). There is also a nucleotide analogue reverse transcriptase inhibitor called tenofovir (*Viread*).

AZT and 3TC is available in a combined pill called *Combivir* and AZT, 3TC and abacavir is available in a combined pill called *Trizivir*.

A single pill combining AZT and abacavir, called *Kivexa* will become available in late 2004/early 2005.

A single pill combining FTC and the nucleotide analogue tenofovir was licensed in the US in the summer of 2004 under the trade name *Truvada*. It should become available in the UK and Europe late in 2004/early 2005.

Non- nucleoside reverse transcriptase inhibitors (NNRTI, or non-Nukes for short)

Drugs in this class include efavirenz (*Sustiva*) and nevirapine (*Viramune*).

Protease inhibitors (PIs)

Drugs in this class include lopinavir/ritonavir (*Kaletra*), indinavir (*Crixivan*), ritonavir (*Norvir*), nelfinavir (*Viracept*), saquinavir hard gel capsules (*Invirase*), saquinavir soft gel capsules (*Fortovase*), atazanavir (*Reyataz*), amprenavir (*Agenerase*), and fosamprenavir (*Telzir*).

Fusion inhibitor

There is only one drug available in this class, T20 (enfuvirtide, *Fuzeon*).

Finding out more

You can find out a lot more about these drugs including by visiting www.aidsmap.com, or by reading the NAM booklet *Anti-HIV drugs*, which is available free of charge from HIV clinics, or can be downloaded from aidsmap.com.

First combination

NNRTI-based

Most British doctors think it is probably best to start with a combination that involves an NNRTI, either efavirenz or nevirapine, taken in combination with two NRTIs. These can be either:

• NNRTI plus AZT/3TC

Or

• NNRTI plus ddI/3TC

Or

• NNRTI plus tenofovir/3TC (if you are coinfected with hepatitis B virus)

Or

• NNRTI plus abacavir/3TC

Several large trials involving thousands of patients have shown that a combination involving efavirenz and AZT/3TC is a first combination which produces very good results, and is most likely to be the first combination you are prescribed.

The reason why doctors and people with HIV prefer this combination is that it has relatively few side-effects and is very easy to take. However, it is very easy to develop resistance to NNRTIs, and if you become resistant to one it's unlikely you'll benefit from using any of the currently available NNRTIs.

Protease inhibitor-based

You can also take a first anti-HIV combination that is based on protease inhibitors. However, if you do take a protease inhibitor as part of your first treatment regimen, it should be a 'boosted' protease inhibitor.

Boosted protease inhibitors include a small dose of the protease inhibitor ritonavir (*Norvir*). There are currently three boosted protease inhibitors in use – *Kaletra* (lopinavir/ritonavir), *Reyataz* (atazanavir/ritonavir) and fosamprenavir (*Telzir*). The addition of the small dose of ritonavir boosts blood levels of the drug, meaning that it has a more powerful anti-HIV effect and you have to take fewer pills, which might make your combination easier to adhere to. However, protease inhibitor-based combinations may involve a greater risk of long-term side-effects and usually involve taking a larger number of pills.

Which nucleosides?

Anti-HIV treatment regimens almost always include two nucleoside/nucleotide analogues. It's not really known which two provide the most effective combination. However, you shouldn't take d4T in your first anti-HIV drug combination because of concerns about side-effects.

The nucleotide analogue tenofovir has been successfully used in initial combinations, and your doctor may be particularly likely to prescribe it if you are infected with hepatitis B virus as well as

HIV, when it should be prescribed with 3TC, which is also effective against hepatitis B.

HIV medicine is evolving very quickly. You can get regular updates on HIV treatments and the best way to use them by visiting www.aidsmap.com. You can also get a free subscription to *AIDS Treatment Update* (ATU), NAM's monthly treatments newsletter, by filling in the form at the back of this book and returning it to the freepost address.

Questions to ask your doctor before starting treatment

What's in the name of a drug?

All medications have at least two names: a generic one, such as zidovudine, and a trade name, such as *Retrovir*, which is used to market the drug and which appears prominently on the packaging, and sometimes on the capsule or tablet itself. Some are also referred to using an abbreviation of their chemical name, e.g. AZT. It is useful to be familiar with all of these names

What does it look like?

If you are trying to decide what medication to take, it may be useful to see the tablets you will have to take. Some people have more difficulty swallowing large pills than others, and if you think the tablets are very large this may cause you difficulties taking them in the future.

The free booklet called *Anti-HIV Drugs* produced by NAM includes pictures of all the drugs and details of the doses, and brief answers to all of the following questions for each drug currently prescribed.

How and when do I need to take it?

Regimens vary from once to four or more times a day, and you may be keen to minimise the number of times you have to take medication each day. Once or twice daily dosing is generally found easier to live with than more frequent dosing. For more information on taking anti-HIV drugs see the chapter *Adherence*.

What side-effects might I experience?

Most drugs will have side-effects, especially during the first few weeks of treatment. If you know what to expect you may find them easier to deal with, or you may decide that you will find a particular type of side-effect particularly bothersome, and would therefore prefer to avoid it. Each drug is associated with different side-effects, but the most common early side-effects tend to be:

- nausea

- headache

- rash

- vomiting

- diarrhoea

- fatigue

Other side-effects may emerge later and may only show up on blood tests, for example:

- tingling in the hands and feet leading to eventual nerve damage (peripheral neuropathy)

- liver toxicities

- neutropenia (low levels of white blood cells needed to fight infections)

- anaemia (low levels of oxygen-bearing red blood cells, leading to tiredness)

- lipodystrophy (changes in body fat) – either fat loss from the face and limbs or fat accumulation in the abdomen and breasts.

Many other side-effects may appear in very small numbers of people. For example, a small number of people who have take protease inhibitors have experienced the onset of diabetes. Because anti-HIV drugs are only tested in a few thousand people before being licensed for widespread use, there is a chance that very rare side-effects will only become apparent when tens of thousands of people have taken the drug.

For more information see the chapter *Side-effects*.

When are the side-effects likely to happen?

Most drug side-effects happen in the first few weeks of treatment as the body adjusts to processing the drug. After a few weeks they begin to get better. Many people report considerable fatigue during the first months of treatment, but it is not clear why this is so.

For more information, see the chapter *Side-effects*.

What can I do to relieve any side-effects I experience?

It is often possible to relieve side-effects by taking other medication which will not interfere with your anti-HIV therapy. For example, your doctor can prescribe anti-nausea drugs and anti-diarrhoea drugs, and painkillers can be used to relieve headaches. Some rashes can be relieved by antihistamines or perhaps steroids, and taking the drugs with food (if recommended) may reduce nausea. However, nothing has yet been discovered to combat the fatigue that may accompany the early stages of a new anti-retroviral regimen, so the only remedy for this is to rest until your energy returns.

Another option with some drugs is to increase the dose gradually.

Is it okay to stop treatment if I can't stand the side-effects, or want a break?

It is best to consult with your doctor before making any changes. You should bear in mind that stopping a drug for more than a few days may mean that you will experience the same side-effects all over again if you resume treatment. Similarly, any gains made in terms of lowering your viral load or raising your CD4 count may be lost quickly whilst you are off treatment.

If you miss doses or reduce the dose rather than stopping treatment altogether, you are likely to increase your risk of developing resistance to one or more of the drugs you are taking (and, potentially, cross-resistance to related drugs that you have not yet taken). However, this varies according to the drugs you are taking. Some drugs leave the body more slowly than others, which is another reason to speak to your doctor beforehand.

Structured treatment interruptions, (the scientific name for treatment breaks) are being investigated by researchers as a means of controlling HIV. However, whether their benefits may outweigh their risks is not yet established. In the meantime, experts are agreed that it is not safe for individuals to experiment with their treatment in this way, unless it is part of a clinical trial.

What can I do if I miss a dose or take too much?

If you miss a single dose by a few hours you should take the missed dose as soon as you can and take the next dose at the normal time. However, if you have missed the dose completely, and only realise this when you come to take the next dose, there is no additional benefit in taking a double dose.

Missed doses are problematic because they lead to falls in drug levels. In turn this can encourage the development of resistance. Missing doses regularly (for example, every weekend) will probably encourage the development of resistance. On the other hand, the occasional missed dose may not cause too many problems.

You may wish to experiment before you start an antiretroviral regimen to see that you can manage it. Try and make it as realistic as possible. If you have several different sorts of low dose vitamin tablets this will be a harmless way of modeling the practice of taking three different drugs at set times each day. Try this for a month and see how you get on. This is a painless way of testing whether you can adhere to a regimen successfully. If you can't manage the regimen you've tested in this way, you may be best advised to look for another one which suits you better.

If you've taken other medication for non-HIV related problems before, don't assume that these will predict your likely adherence to combination therapy. Any medication which prevents the immediate recurrence of a condition is likely to be taken more consistently than one where the effect of non-compliance is only visible through laboratory tests.

For more information see the chapter *Adherence*.

Will anti-HIV drugs interact with other drugs I take?

Anti-HIV drugs, particularly protease inhibitors, interact with many other drugs including prescription drugs, over-the-counter drugs, recreational drugs and herbal preparations. Drug interactions may cause serious side-effects. Furthermore, interactions may mean that one or more of your medicines don't work properly.

Do I need to take the drugs on a full or empty stomach?

The absorption of some drugs can be seriously affected by the presence of absence of food in the stomach. For these drugs you will be instructed to take your medication with or without food as necessary.

Are there any foods I should avoid?

You should be given detailed instructions about what you should and shouldn't eat when taking this medication. Fortunately, the restrictions on food relate more to whether you should take drugs on a full stomach or not rather than whether you should avoid food.

Do I need to be careful about drinking or recreational drug use on this treatment?

Very few anti-HIV drugs are affected by alcohol, although the pancreatitis risk of some drugs, such as ddI, may be increased if you drink heavily, in the view of some doctors. Pancreatitis and peripheral neuropathy are in any case associated with heavy alcohol consumption. Alcohol may also affect your liver's capacity to process antiretroviral drugs, and may increase nausea.

For information about anti-HIV drugs and recreational drugs see the chapter *Daily health issues.*

What do I do if I think I am pregnant or want to become pregnant?

If you are already on treatment, any potential adverse effects of drugs on your baby are most likely to occur during the first 14 weeks of pregancy. HIV transmission is more likely to occur during delivery, but transmission has been shown to occur during the first 14 weeks of pregancy, so the option of stopping treatment needs to be balanced against the potential risk of a rebound in viral load if you come off treatment. Increased viral load increases the risk of HIV transmission from mother-to-child.

If you want to conceive you should discuss the relative risks of coming off treatment or conceiving whilst on treatment with your doctor.

For more information see *Mother-to-baby transmission of HIV.*

Do I need to think about taking time off work while my body gets used to these drugs?

Some people find that it may take several weeks before they feel well enough to go back to work, or before they can manage without childcare assistance, when they begin anti-HIV treatment.

Do these drugs need to be kept in the fridge or in a special container?

Some drugs may deteriorate in hot conditions and so may require refrigeration, or to be stored in a cool place, out of direct sunlight. Other drugs may be affected by damp conditions, e.g. indinavir. This drug must be kept in a container with a special dessicant (a susbtance which draws moisture out of the air) and shouldn't be kept in a box with other pills, or in the fridge. Your doctor or pharmacist will be able to provide advice on this.

Can I take them on holiday?

The major difficulty with taking these drugs on holiday is the number of containers you may have to carry and the attention this may draw to your HIV-positive status. However, none of the packaging for these drugs reveals that they are prescribed for the treatment of HIV infection, and a letter from your doctor which says that you are prescribed these specific drugs should provide sufficient cover for you. Difficulty may come for people who wish to enter the United States however, where entry for HIV-positive people is restricted.

If you are going to a hot climate lopinavir, ritonavir and saquinavir may deteriorate because of the heat, and indinavir may deteriorate because of humidity. Be sure to keep indinavir capsules in a dry place, and keep them in the original container with the dessicant supplied as far as possible.

Alterations in time zones and the eating schedules (and size of portions!) on long-haul flights may be more problematic. People who work on airlines tend to keep to the time zone of their home country wherever they are working, but this is more difficult for people who are travelling somewhere for several days or weeks. Although airlines recommend that you switch into the time zone of your destination as soon as the flight begins (in order to combat jet lag), this may be confusing if you are trying to stick to a schedule. Eight or 12 hour changes in time zones are likely to be relatively easy to work with; shorter or longer adjustments (from Europe to the Middle East, Latin America, the East Coast of the United States, India, Australia and the Pacific) may be more problematic.

If you are gone for less than five days, it will probably work out easier to stick to home time, but if you are away for longer, try to tailor your dosing times to the time zone of your destination as quickly as possible without missing doses (remember that with most drugs you have a couple of hours leeway either side of the

12 hour or 8 hour intervals at which you are meant to take the drugs).

For more information see the chapters *Adherence* and *Travel*.

Should I drive a car or operate machinery while taking these drugs?

If any medication is causing drowsiness, dizziness, loss of concentration or fatigue you should be very careful about driving or operating machinery. These have all been reported as early side-effects of some antiretroviral drugs.

How can I get further information about this treatment if I want it?

A variety of sources can provide you with information about the treatment prescribed to you, but at the very least your doctor should provide you with a clear explanation of any of the issues discussed in this section, supported by written information to take home. Some drug companies have produced information booklets about their drugs which may answer some of these questions, but if your doctor is not available, the first port of call may be your HIV pharmacist, who should know the answers to all the questions discussed in this section. Your doctor should provide you with information on where to go if you have any questions on your treatment.

Changing treatment due to failure

As mentioned above, the goal of anti-HIV treatment, if you are taking it for the first time, is to reduce your viral load to below the limit of detection, which, using current tests, is 50 copies/ml. If your viral load doesn't fall below this level, then it's more likely that your treatments won't suppress HIV for long.

If your viral load falls below 50, then rebounds to above 50 on two consecutive tests, then it means that your treatment is failing. You may find that your CD4 cell count starts to fall, which will mean that your risk of becoming ill because of HIV increases.

If your treatment fails to get your viral load below 50, or it rebounds above this level, then there's a possible risk that you will develop resistance to some or all of the anti-HIV drugs you are taking.

If your treatment is not suppressing your viral load to undetectable levels, it should be changed.

Occasionally, your viral load may rise a little above 50 before dropping down to undetectable levels on the next test. These changes are called 'blips' and mean that you should have your viral load retested as soon as possible. Blips are often due to a problem with the testing equipment, but could be a warning sign of other problems, such as treatment failure, drug interactions, poor adherence or illness.

If you have two viral load tests at least a month apart and both show that your viral load is above 400, then a treatment change should be considered. It's recommended that you have a resistance test to see which of your drugs isn't working and to help you choose replacement drugs. These tests are only accurate if your viral load is above 1,000, and if you change drugs due to treatment failure without having a resistance test, it's recommended that your new treatment regimen consists of a completely new set of drugs.

If you have to change treatments because of side-effects and have an undetectable viral load, then it's completely safe to only switch the drug or drugs causing the problem.

Anti-HIV drugs have to be taken very consistently to work properly (this is called adherence), so if you haven't been taking your treatment properly for any reason, make sure that you switch to a new combination which is easier to take, and fits in with the way you live your life.

Changing treatment due to lipodystrophy

Lipodystrophy is the name given to a syndrome of side-effects caused by anti-HIV drugs. It includes an increase in fats in the blood (which can increase your long-term risk of a heart attack, diabetes and stroke), and changes in body shape (including fat loss from the face, limbs and buttocks), and fat gain (at the back of the neck – sometimes called buffalo hump – and around the stomach).

The NRTI d4T has been particularly associated with fat loss, and if you are taking d4T you are recommended to switch it for another drug, if you have treatment options available.

If you have high blood fats and are taking a protease inhibitor, then it might be worth switching to an NNRTI, if this option is available to you. Changes in your diet can also help, see the chapter *Nutrition and HIV*. Exercise can also be helpful and is looked at in more detail in the chapter *Exercise*. Your doctor can also prescribe drugs (called statin and fibrates) to control fats in your blood.

Changing your treatment appears to have only a very minimal impact on body fat changes. Lost fat has been shown to slowly return to the limbs for two years after switching from d4T to abacavir. Fat loss can be very distressing, particularly fat loss from the face. The use of a cosmetic treatment called *New Fill* (polylactic acid) can help fill out the checks and remedy the wasted appearance that facial fat loss causes. Treatment involves a course of injections, and it may have to be repeated. Some, but not all, HIV clinics provide the treatment for free on the NHS, but some people have to obtain *New Fill* treatment privately. A single course of treatment costs from £800 – £1,200.

Surgery is sometimes used to remove fat which has accumulated around the back of the neck.

Fat loss and fat gain caused by anti-HIV drugs can be very emotionally distressing and uncomfortable. It's important that you let your doctor know how body fat changes are affecting you. If you have fat loss from the face or fat gain around the neck, your doctor may be able to refer you for cosmetic surgery to help correct it. Staff at hospitals with large HIV clinics are becoming very skilled at providing cosmetic treatments for fat loss and fat gain caused by anti-HIV drugs. Also make sure that you tell your doctor if changes in your body shape are causing emotional or psychological problems, as mental health support will be available.

Salvage therapy

If you are resistant to many anti-HIV drugs from more than one drug class, then you might find it harder to assemble a drug regimen which will get your viral load down to undetectable levels.

But it's still worth taking anti-HIV treatment. Even if your treatments are unable to achieve an undetectable viral load, your health is still likely to benefit. If you have limited treatment options, your CD4 cell count might be a better tool to assess the effectiveness of your treatment. Finding a new treatment regimen that will increase your CD4 cell count, your health, and your quality of life is likely to be a better option than trying to assemble a combination to control your viral load.

If you are resistant to drugs from all three main classes of anti-HIV drugs (NRTIs, NNRTIs and protease inhibitors), doctors often say you need 'salvage therapy'.

The more new drugs you can add to a combination, the more likely it is that your salvage regimen will work. Resistance tests should be used to help determine which drugs will work best for you. Tests to measure the amount of anti-HIV drugs in your blood may also be useful to ensure that you are taking the most effective dose of your medication.

Use of T-20

T-20 (enfuvirtide, *Fuzeon*) belongs to a new class of anti-HIV drugs called fusion inhibitors, and has been licensed for use in people who have very few treatment options. Unlike all the other anti-HIV drugs, T-20 needs to be injected, twice daily under the skin.

T-20 achieves the best results if you can take it along with other anti-HIV drugs that still work for you. If you are taking T-20 and it is the only anti-HIV drug that you are sensitive to, then you'll rapidly develop resistance to it. But even in these circumstances, it might prove to have some benefit.

Treatment breaks

There's a lot of discussion about the value and safety of taking a supervised break from your HIV treatments (called a structured treatment interruption).

Doctors had hoped that taking structured treatment breaks would help to prime the immune system to control HIV without the use of anti-HIV drugs. Studies have shown that this is not the case.

However, another reason why some people are interested in them is the opportunity they may give individuals to take a break from anti-HIV treatment and its side-effects.

The potential benefits of a structured treatment interruption are a boosted immune system and fewer side-effects.

However, structured treatment breaks are not without risks. Some people have reported complications, including a rapid fall in their CD4 cell count, illness due to HIV and the development of more drug resistance.

If you are considering taking a break from your treatment, make sure that you discuss it carefully with your doctor beforehand.

Don't take a break from your treatment if your CD4 cell count is below 200 – there's a very real risk that you could develop a very serious infection.

If your lowest ever CD4 cell count was below 200 you are at higher risk of developing AIDS-defining illnesses during a treatment break.

Further reading

NAM factsheets, *Anti-HIV therapy*, *Changing treatment* and *Treatment interruption*.

Anti-HIV drugs, Clinical trials, HIV therapy and *Lipodystrophy*, booklets in the information for HIV-positive people series produced by NAM.

'Anti-HIV therapy' in NAM's *HIV and AIDS Treatments Directory*.

African men and combination therapy, African women and combination therapy, Gay men and combination therapy and *Decisions*, leaflets produced by the Terrence Higgins Trust.

Starting treatment – by Christopher

Following my HIV diagnosis in August 2001, my doctor estimated that I would be looking to start therapy in around six years. But following a rapid CD4 cell decline, it was only nine months later that he suggested I start thinking about choosing a drug regimen.

It's an understatement to say that I was disappointed with the way things had gone. I'd spent the previous year or so trying to find out as much as I could about HIV and its treatment – as a pharmacologist working in a university laboratory I felt at home with the scientific and clinical literature and was encouraged by what I had seen.

But when the imminence of my own HAART debut was staring me in the face, my level-headedness flew out of the window. It was like a second diagnosis. I was really scared.

For the next year or so, I regularly visited a treatments adviser at the clinic. She talked me through the various drug options available to me, and we eventually decided on a regimen of efavirenz and *Combivir*. While I was aware of the potential neuropsychiatric side-effects of efavirenz, protease inhibitors – particularly the threat of lipodystrophy – terrified me.

The year or so of two-monthly visits to the clinic were an exercise in procrastination. Every time I went back, I produced another excuse for delaying therapy – while they seemed genuine reasons to me at the time, it's clear to me now that I was avoiding facing up to my predicament. So, while my CD4 count hovered around the 200 mark, my adviser's patience eventually began to wear thin. Eventually my excuses ran out and, armed with a carrier bag full of pills, I reluctantly fixed a date to start.

I took my first *Combivir* pill during a coffee break at work. I spent the next four hours gazing out of my office window, waiting for the nausea to kick in, or to be rushing to the toilet with diarrhoea. They never came.

In the evening, I swallowed my first dose of efavirenz along with my second *Combivir* pill, half-expecting hellish nightmares and night sweats or suicidal feelings in the morning. After sleeping like a baby, I spent the next day feeling a little like I had smoked a joint in the morning – precisely as my adviser had warned me I would. The feeling was far from unpleasant.

The stoned feeling had worn off by the end of the day, and the morning grogginess disappeared entirely within three days. I tentatively started drinking alcohol again a few days later, with no unexpected effects, and rekindled my nocturnal dancing habits within two weeks – to find that "the efavirenz feeling", rather than forcing me to curtail my nights out, had added an interesting twist to the 4am taxi ride home.

I've now been on my combination for 18 months. It reduced my viral load to undetectable levels immediately, although its effects on my CD4 count took almost a year to kick in. Now, my CD4 count is marching up at a respectable pace, and I'm still free of side-effects.

Sure, I sometimes have diarrhoea, and I've had a bout of distressing nightmares recently. It's all too easy to put these down to the drugs and feel sorry for myself. But I try to remember that I've always had diarrhoea occasionally, and I remember worse dreams from my pre-HAART days.

My only regret is that I didn't start HAART little earlier, to increase my chances of a sustainable response to my current and future drug regimens – my CD4 count dipped below 200 on more occasions than I would like while I procrastinated. But at the time I didn't have the benefit of hindsight, so now the best I can do is enjoy these side-effect-free years, and hope that my next combinations will be as easy as my first.

Finally undetectable! by Edwin

After almost 15 years of HIV, and six years of viral load testing, I heard on Thursday, June 21st 2001 that my viral load had dropped to an undetectable level for the first time. It was a milestone neither I nor my HIV consultant ever expected me to reach.

Fifteen months earlier I had taken a planned treatment interruption, and went off all antiretrovirals for a year. I had been on a variety of treatments, beginning with AZT monotherapy, since 1993. When the HAART era began, I had already become resistant to protease inhibitors, due to suboptimal early dosing of saquinavir, and by 1999 I was resistant to all three classes of currently available drugs. My liver also needed to recover from a (mitochondrially) toxic d4T/3TC combo.

Taking the treatment break wasn't an easy decision, but with my liver about to explode, apparently, and a rising viral load, there seemed to be little choice. I kept going with acupuncture and herbs, managed a once-in-a-lifetime Millennium trip to Australia, and then, once my viral load began to hit the half-million mark, slowly began to fade.

I used all of what little energy I had to read everything about the latest treatments, including everything from NAM, and reviewed all my resistance tests. In February 2000, Kaletra (lopinavir/ritonavir) became available in Canada (where I was living at the time) on expanded access. Together with my HIV consultant, we settled on restarting with five drugs, recycling several older options, and including a completely experimental drug called mycophenolate.

Amazingly, my liver didn't explode, and although I had the usual nausea and diarrhoea associated with starting a new regimen, within a few weeks I felt human again. After a month, my viral load plummeted from over 600,000 to the 5,000 range. My CD4s began to slowly increase, but I decided to try and throw everything at the virus in order to give me the best chance of a full immune recovery.

A few months later, during a holiday in Spain, I added another three drugs, making eight in total. I was nervous adding more away from home, but since I was British, I naively figured I could get free hospital treatment in Spain if there were problems. Fortunately there weren't, and, frustratingly, my viral load settled, remaining between 100-500 for the rest of 2000.

I was one of the first to be offered therapeutic drug level monitoring in early 2001, and we discovered that all my measurable drug levels were far too low, despite above-average doses of Kaletra. My viral load finally reached undetectable after further adjustments,and another day of therapeutic drug monitoring.

From being at death's door in March 2000, with a CD4 count of 30, I felt like I got my life back by the summer of 2001, with 210 CD4s. Most amazingly, my liver function tests were completely normal.

Therapeutic drug monitoring, along with Virtual Genotype testing, a great consultant, great GP, amazing partner and, above all, an almost pathological determination to beat HIV, got me to that point. Today my viral load is still undetectable and I'm taking 'only' six different antiretrovirals and two lipid-lowering pills as well as testosterone injections in order to live a full and happy life!

If anyone tells you that all that is left is palliative care and you're not ready, or you are too frightened to try new treatments, don't give up. For me, at least, the fight was worth it.

Robert and treatment

I was diagnosed HIV-positive in 1997. I'm now 65. It was a bit of a shock. It could neverhappen to me, after all. I only found out because of someone's kindness and honesty.

In the autumn of 1997, I had felt really out-of-sorts; I developed 'flu (which I'd never had before) and came out in a rash – which I now know was probably the HIV starting. I got over that, but still felt awful. The "someone" kept asking me to go over, as he wanted to tell me something "important", but I just didn't feel up to it.

Anyway, eventually I did go, and he said something like "I've something to tell you." He said that he had been diagnosed HIV-positive on his annual test. So I had "the test" too, and learned that I was HIV-positive.

My blood tests showed that my viral load was 500,000 and my CD4 cell count was 210! I was put on anti-HIV drugs immediately. The drugs were indinavir, AZT, and ddI. I hated the regime because of indinavir, and its eating restrictions. Anyway, I carried on enthusiastically with my job as a lecturer in computing subjects at a local college of further education.

Side-effects developed, though my viral load came down to 'undetectable' in six months and my CD4 count went up to 400. I became very weak in my legs – I could hardly climb onto a stool, or get up if I was lying sunbathing! Also, my cholesterol level went up sharply, which was actually the saving of me!

The clinic altered my treatment because of the rise in my cholesterol levels, replacing the indinavir with efavirenz.

What a relief! No restrictions, and all my strength came back. I don't 'work out', but always do sensible things like cycling a bit, walking, eating well (and enjoying wine and beer). I don't take drugs or smoke.

Eventually, a job was advertised for a network manager for a nearby comprehensive school, and, again being very positive in my life attitude, I applied, and was accepted. I didn't disclose my HIV status, only my GP knows it. At first just me, my team has grown, and I love it!! I've been doing the job for over five years now.

I am a very happy sort of person, and hardly think of my HIV status. I just take the tablets (never missing a dose) and get on with my life. My viral load is still undetectable.

As Woody Allen said, 'It's not that I'm afraid to die, I just don't want to be there when it happens.'

Adherence

Introduction

Taking your anti-HIV medication properly is the single most important thing you can do to ensure the success of your anti-HIV treatments.

Adherence to your anti-HIV treatments involves the following elements:

• Taking all the drugs that make up your anti-HIV treatment regimen.

• Taking the right number of pills.

• Taking your drugs the correct number of times each day.

• Taking your drugs at the right time – (taking your medicines too late, or too early can be as bad as not taking them at all).

• Taking your drugs with or without food according to instructions.

• Making sure that your drugs don't interact with other medicines prescribed to you, or bought over the counter. Herbal remedies and recreational drugs can also interact with anti-HIV medication.

Why adherence is important

Not taking your HIV medications properly can mean that they do not work effectively, leading to an increase in your viral load, a fall in your CD4 cell count and a greater risk of becoming ill and dying because of HIV.

The reason adherence is so important is because HIV can quickly become resistant to the drugs used to treat it. If the blood level of an anti-HIV drug drops too low, then it will be unable to stop HIV reproducing and this gives the virus an opportunity to develop resistance. The drug-resistant strains of the virus will become dominant.

This could mean that not only do you become resistant to the drugs you are currently taking, but also to drugs similar to these. For example, if you develop resistance to one NNRTI, you're likely to become resistant to all NNRTIs. This is called cross-resistance, and although the risk varies from drug to drug, cross-resistance can occur in all classes of drug used to treat HIV.

Adherence is so important that many doctors think it is better to stop treatment altogether rather than miss doses. However, this carries it own risks, and if you are finding it difficult to take your medication and think that you need a break from your treatment, discuss the pros and cons with your doctor.

Level of adherence to aim for

You should try and take all your doses correctly. The best response to anti-HIV therapy is seen in people who had 100% adherence to their treatment. Levels of adherence of less than 95% have been associated with poor suppression of HIV viral load, rebound in viral load, and either poor CD4 cell gains or falls in CD4 cell count.

If you are taking your treatment once a day, 95% adherence means missing, or incorrectly taking, only one dose a month.

If you are taking your treatment twice a day, 95% adherence means missing, or incorrectly taking, only three doses a month.

If you are taking your medication three times a day, 95% adherence means missing, or incorrectly taking, only four doses a month.

Adherence at this level can be very hard, and is much higher than the level needed for other medication. Nevertheless, try to take all your doses. Remember, any fall in the level of drug levels in your blood will give an opportunity for strains of HIV to develop which drugs don't work against.

How to boost your chances of adherence

You are more likely to adhere to your HIV treatments if you were involved in the decisions both to start treatment and about which drugs to start treatment with.

Being honest about your lifestyle to yourself and your doctor can help ensure that you start on a combination that is right for you. Don't make unrealistic demands on yourself, and think about how taking medication will fit in with your social, working, eating and sleeping patterns. The chances are that there will be a combination available that will mean that you don't have to change your lifestyle at all, or make only modest alterations to your routine.

Side-effects are a very common reason why people skip doses. If you are experiencing side-effects of any kind, make sure you tell your doctor. The chances are that there will be another treatment option available. It's better to change treatments than miss doses and risk resistance.

Taking handfuls of pills is often cited by people as a reason why they miss doses. Doctors call the number of pills you have to take your 'pill burden'. If you find taking lots of pills a problem, then talk to your doctor about taking a combination with as few pills as possible. It might be that you can switch to a combination that involves taking no more than a couple of pills twice a day. But make sure that you consider how these 'easy to take' regimens fit in with the reality of your day-to-day life.

Depression and other emotional and mental health problems have been linked with low levels of adherence. If you're depressed and don't think that you can cope with starting HIV treatments, then it might be best to wait until you feel more able to cope.

Similarly, if you become depressed whilst taking treatments, it's important to seek help. Depression is very common in people with HIV (see the chapter on *Mental health*), and many HIV clinics have specialist mental health teams who can offer treatment and support. Treatments for depression work just as well in HIV-positive people.

Having problems with money and housing, and feeling isolated have also been known to be associated with low levels of adherence in some people. Many HIV organisations can provide advice about money and accommodation, and your HIV clinic may even have a specialist HIV social worker you can see for advice. If you have family or friends who know that you are taking HIV-medication, try and talk to them about the problems you are experiencing – you might find that they are able to offer wonderful support. On the other hand, if you are worried about people close to you knowing that you have HIV, you might find that one solution is an adherence support group involving other HIV-positive people. These are organised by many HIV clinics and HIV support agencies.

Late doses

Taking your medication too late (or too early) can be as bad as not taking it at all, and can allow HIV to become resistant to some or all of the drugs you are taking.

The safest approach is to aim to take all your medicines at the right time and in the right way. But, being honest, there are bound to be times when you take your medicine late. As long as this happens very occasionally, it shouldn't make any difference to the success of your treatments. However, regularly taking your medication late or early will give HIV an opportunity to become resistant.

Not all anti-HIV drugs are processed by the body at the same rate. Protease inhibitors, particularly those that aren't boosted by a small dose of ritonavir, are metabolised very rapidly, meaning that it's particularly important to take them correctly.

Other drugs, for example NNRTIs, are more forgiving and it's not quite so important to take them at very strict intervals – taking them an hour or so late shouldn't make too much of a difference.

Don't assume that because somebody else has taken their anti-HIV drugs constantly late and still has an undetectable viral load, that this will be the case for you, even if they are taking the same drugs as you. The speed and efficiency with which individuals process medicines can vary a lot.

If the way you live your life means that you find it very hard to stick to strict dosing schedules, then talk to your doctor about the possibility of switching to a more 'forgiving' combination.

Should you forget to take a dose of your drugs, take it as soon as you remember, and then carry on with your normal dosing schedule. Don't take a double dose to make up for the one you missed.

You might find that breaking your routine in some way increases the chances that you forget to take your pills on time. If you know that your normal dosing schedule is going to be disrupted, then try and make a plan that ensures you take your medication properly. If you do forget to take your dose, don't beat yourself up, but try and learn from it so it doesn't happen again.

Support from your clinic

If you understand why you are taking HIV treatment and why adherence is important, then you're more likely to take your treatments properly.

When you are first prescribed anti-HIV drugs, your doctor should explain when and how to take them. You should also be given written information to take away and read. This should help you to remember what the doctor told you.

You should also be told what side-effects to expect. Most HIV drugs cause unwanted side-effects, but on the whole these tend to be mild and go away over time. Knowing what to expect might make the side-effects easier to plan for and cope with. This should mean that you are more likely to think that they are worth getting through and so continue to take your medication.

In summary, when you first begin or, if you need to, change treatments you should understand:

- Why you have been given these drugs.

- How often you need to take them.

- If there are any dietary restrictions.

- If there are any side-effects and how to manage them (and when to seek urgent medical advice).

- Where you can get help and advice (including during normal working hours and at the evenings and weekends. Many hospitals have a 24-hour pharmacy support line).

Taking anti-HIV medication is likely to be a life-long commitment, and you may find that you need different levels of adherence support at different times. Make sure that you tell a doctor, nurse or pharmacist if you are having problems with adherence. They shouldn't judge you and will almost certainly be able to help.

Adherence tips

Simple forgetfulness is probably the most common reason why people miss doses of anti-HIV drugs. Don't give yourself too hard a time if this happens occasionally – you're only human, after all. But if it's happening often, talk to your doctor about it. It might be that you can change to a treatment combination that is easier to adhere to. If this isn't an option, then there might be some practical support that can be offered to help you manage your treatment better.

It could be that you just need a few prompts or reminders to boost your adherence. Listed below are a few strategies you might find useful.

Practice

Before you start taking a combination, if possible, practice for a few weeks before. For example, take sweets or multivitamins in the same quantities and at the same time as you would have to take your anti-HIV drugs. Make sure that you also follow any dietary restrictions.

Keep a diary

Have a written record of the doses you need to take. Tick off each dose as you take it. You can download a drug diary from the factsheets section at www.aidsmap.com.

Jog your memory

If you need a reminder, then setting an alarm on a watch might prove useful.

Pill boxes

You can get partitioned containers from your clinic to fill every week or few days with individual doses. Keep doses in different places where you might be when the time you need to take a dose comes around, for example at work, in your bag, or at a friend's house. Make sure that the container is suitable – pills can deteriorate if not stored properly – and remember that medicines have a use-by date. Make sure that you store medicines out of the reach of children, and avoid places that are very cold or hot.

Holidays, travel, and going out

Going away on holiday can have an effect on your adherence. Travelling long distances might disrupt your medicine schedule. Make sure that you take enough medicine with you, and always travel with your pills in your hand luggage. That way, it's closer to hand if you need to take it during your journey and is also less likely to get lost.

Holidays involve a break in routine, which could mean that you miss some of the prompts that remind you to take your drugs. It may help if you think in advance of other ways to remember them.

Taking your medicine away from home may mean that you will have to take it around people who don't know about your health, or whom you don't want to know. Plan in advance how to manage this. Simple things like having a bottle of water by your bed, and a handy snack like a chocolate bar, might give you the privacy you need to take your medicines.

Even going out for the evening can increase the chances that you might miss a dose. So make sure that you have any necessary medicine on you before you leave home. If you're going to a club and are likely to be searched, there's a chance that door staff might not recognise prescription medicines. There have been cases of people having their HIV medication confiscated by bouncers when trying to get into clubs.

Simply having a good time, particularly if you've been drinking or taking drugs, can also increase your chances of missing a dose. Try and have a prompt to remind you to take your medicines. Also remember that anti-HIV drugs and recreational drugs can interact. Ask your doctor or other member of your healthcare team if this is a concern for you. They should be able to offer advice about minimising the risk. Don't skip doses.

Further reading

NAM factsheets, *Adherence, Adherence tips, Drug diary, Drug check-list* and *Late doses*

Adherence, booklet produced by NAM.

'Anti-HIV therapy' in NAM's *HIV and AIDS Treatments Directory.*

Things to help you stick with it, leaflet produced by the Terrence Higgins Trust.

Side-effects

Introduction

Nearly every medicine can cause unwanted side-effects in some people.

Side-effects are a common cause of illness, discomfort and distress in people taking anti-HIV drugs – even people who have an undetectable viral load and high CD4 cell count and don't have any symptoms of HIV infection.

However, it's not inevitable that you will experience side-effects from any of the medicines you are given to fight HIV or other infections. It's also worth remembering that a lot of side-effects are mild, can be controlled with other medicines, and lessen or even go away over time.

Types of side-effects

There are two main reasons for side-effects: an allergic reaction to the drug which causes side-effects, or side-effects caused by the direct effects of a medicine.

An allergic reaction will cause side-effects such as a rash or fever. You should contact your doctor immediately if you suspect that you have developed an allergic reaction to any medicine you are taking. An allergic (hypersensitivity) reaction to abacavir (*Ziagen*) can be potentially fatal. If you are taking abacavir you should read carefully the warning card that comes with boxes of the medicines and contact your doctor immediately if you experience any symptoms suggesting that you might be experiencing an allergic reaction to the drug.

If a side-effect is being caused by the unwanted effects of a drug itself, the nature of the side-effect might depend on which part of the body the drug is intended to treat, or the way in which the body processes the drug. For example, some drugs can damage the cells in bone marrow which are responsible for producing new blood cells, so this could mean that your body doesn't produce enough red or white blood cells. Some medicines can make you feel generally unwell, or cause vomiting, nausea, or diarrhoea. Reduced sex drive or sexual problems are another common side-effect.

Side-effects are often related to the amount of drug you are taking – for some drugs, but not all, it is possible to adjust the dose you receive to help mininise the risk of side-effects.

When side-effects develop

Side-effects soon after starting treatment

Most side-effects occur after you have been taking a medicine for a week or two. However, there is no strict pattern, and some people develop side-effects after taking their first dose of a drug. For others, side-effects don't develop for many months.

Side-effects occur in the first month or so of taking a drug not because you are being poisoned by the medicine, but because you have especially high concentrations of a drug in your blood in the weeks and months after you first start taking it. Over time, the peak drug levels in your blood go down, and side-effects tend to wear off. Because of this, it might be recommended in some cases that you gradually increase the dose you take of a drug over a few weeks.

Side-effects are often worse during the first month or so of taking a drug. Over time, they may lessen, modify, or go away altogether.

Daily pattern to side-effects

There can be a daily pattern to side-effects, linked to the time you take your medicines and also to the processing of the drug by your body. It might be possible to minimise the inconvenience that this causes by adjusting the time at which you take your medicines. For example, the NNRTI efavirenz (*Sustiva*) can cause dizziness and other psychological side-effects. Many people overcome these by taking their daily dose of the drug just before going to bed.

Medicines to control side-effects

Medicines are available to help control side-effects in both the short and the long term. These include anti-sickness and anti-diarrhoea drugs.

Longer-term side-effects

It's also known that some side-effects only develop in the longer-term. For example, lipodystrophy, changes in body shape and blood fats, has been seen in people taking anti-HIV drugs for a number of months or years. A rare, but serious long-term side-effect is called lactic acidosis. There's a lot more information about lipodystrophy later in this chapter.

Side-effects and a weakened immune system

If you have a very weak immune system there's some evidence to suggest that you might be more vulnerable to side-effects, including painful nerve damage to the feet (peripheral neuropathy) and fat loss from the face, when you start taking anti-HIV drugs if your immune system is already severely damaged by HIV. There's a lot more information about peripheral neuropathy later in this chapter.

Coping with side-effects

The risk of side-effects might be something you consider when deciding whether or not to take a certain treatment. If you are ill, or at risk of becoming ill, the benefits of the treatment may well be clear-cut and far outweigh the risk of side-effects.

If you have decided it is worthwhile taking a treatment and you do develop side-effects, it's important to establish which drug is causing the problem. This can be quite tricky if you are taking anti-HIV medication, as more than one of the drugs might have the potential to cause the side-effects you are experiencing.

Talk about problems you are experiencing with side-effects with your doctor. Don't stop taking treatments without seeking medical advice.

Taking other medicines, such as anti-sickness or anti-nausea medication, can help control side-effects.

If it's known that a particular anti-HIV drug is causing side-effects, then there's a good chance, particularly if you've never taken anti-HIV drugs before, that you will be able to switch to a drug that doesn't cause the side-effects you are experiencing.

Nausea, lipodystrophy and peripheral neuropathy

Three common and distressing side-effects of anti-HIV treatment are nausea, lipodystrophy (changes in body shape and increased blood lipids) and peripheral neuropathy (painful damage to the nerves in the feet, lower legs and, sometimes, the hands). Detailed information on these side-effects is provided below.

Nausea and vomiting

Many anti-HIV drugs are associated with nausea. However, it is most commonly reported as a side-effect of AZT (zidovudine, *Retrovir*), d4T (stavudine, *Sustiva*), 3TC (lamivudine, *Epivir*), and abacavir (*Ziagen*) from the NRTI class. Protease inhibitors which commonly cause nausea include indinavir (*Crixivan*) and ritonavir (*Norvir*) and those containing a small dose of ritonavir to boost their effectiveness. Some of the drugs used to treat infections commonly seen in people with HIV also cause nausea, including cidofovir, foscarnet, ganciclovir, intravenous pentamidine, co-trimoxazole and clarithronycin.

If nausea is accompanied by other symptoms, the underlying cause needs to be investigated and treated. If it is due to drug side-effects, then the dose and frequency may need to be altered or the drug discontinued. For example, the nausea and vomiting which can accompany use of the protease inhibitor ritonavir may be eased by splitting the usual daily dose, i.e. changing from 600mg or 7.5ml twice daily to 300mg or 3.75ml four times daily. This would result in less extreme variations in the concentration of ritonavir in the bloodstream and body tissues. Don't alter the dosing of your treatments without discussing it with your doctor first.

Some drugs, e.g. AZT, can be taken with food in order to limit nausea. Talk to your HIV pharmacist or doctor about this to clarify which foods can be eaten with your medication, and which to avoid, or see *Nutrition* in NAM's information series for people with HIV.

Anti-nausea medication

Anti-nausea medication (sometimes called anti-emetics), taken either as tablets or injections, can be prescribed by your doctor to help manage symptoms. This can be particularly important when starting a new treatment, such as anti-HIV combination therapy, which is associated with a high risk of nausea and vomiting during the first few weeks. Adequate anti-nausea medication can help you adjust to your new regimen and make this initial period easier.

Many different drugs are used to treat nausea and/or vomiting. These include metoclopramide, prochlorperazine, perphenazine, trifluoperazine, chlorpromazine, domperidone, granisetron, ondansetron, tropisetron and nabilone.

Coping with nausea and vomiting

For some people, having to swallow large tablets or large numbers of tablets can itself bring on bouts of nausea. If you think this might be a problem for you, it might influence your choice of anti-HIV therapy. For example, you could ask to see the different drugs available and find out about the number of doses required.

Whatever the cause, do not feel obliged to "grin and bear it" – nausea and vomiting can prevent you from getting enough food and nutrients and from sticking with your chosen treatment regimen. As well as asking your doctor about anti-emetic medication, the following practical tips may be helpful and can be discussed with an HIV dietitian:

- Eat small, frequent meals throughout the day rather than two or three large meals.

- Don't eat liquid and solid food at the same meal. Space them at least one hour apart.

- Avoid eating greasy, fatty, fried or spicy food. Instead, choose bland food.

- Try dry food such as toast, crackers, cereal, and fruit and vegetables that are bland or soft.

- Salty food such as crackers, pretzels and popcorn can help reduce nausea. Carry a packet with you when you leave the house.

- Don't lie flat for at least an hour after you eat.

- Eat food cold or at room temperature – hot food can worsen nausea.

- Herbal tea (e.g. peppermint or chamomile) or root ginger can help settle upset stomachs.

Lipodystropy

Changes in body shape and the metabolism caused by anti-HIV drugs are known as lipodystrophy. Only a minority of people who take anti-HIV drugs develop lipodystrophy.

Changes in body shape

Three different patterns of body fat change have been seen in people taking anti-HIV drugs. These are:

- Fat gain on the abdomen/belly, between the shoulder blades, around the neck, or in the breasts.

- Fat loss from under the skin which is most noticeable in the arms and legs, buttocks, and face, causing prominent veins in the limbs, shrunken buttocks, and facial wasting.

- A mixture of both fat gain and fat loss.

The fat gain in the belly which some people develop isn't made up of fat under the skin. Rather, it is caused by the build-up of fat within the abdomen. This makes the belly feel harder.

The majority of people who develop these changes experience a combination of both fat loss and fat gain, and you may often hear these body shape changes described as 'fat redistribution'.

A few people may also develop small, isolated fat deposits, called lipomas. Typically, these occur in the trunk and limbs.

Changes in body shape can be accompanied by changes in the body's metabolism.

The risk of developing body shape changes

It's not known exactly who will develop body shape changes whilst taking anti-HIV drugs. However, it seems that the risk is increased if:

- You take a combination of anti-HIV drugs including protease inhibitors and NRTIs, especially d4T (stavudine, *Zerit*).

- You start taking anti-HIV drugs when you have a very low CD4 cell count.

It also seems that the following factors may increase your risk of body fat changes developing:

- Studies have shown that the longer you take anti-HIV drugs, the greater your risk of body fat changes occurring. One study showed that after three years of taking a combination which included a protease inhibitor and NRTIs, between 30%-40% of people developed some kind of body fat change. It's not known if the risk carries on growing after this point or if people who are likely to develop lipodystrophy will have done so by this point.

• People who are overweight seem more likely to develop central fat accumulation.

• Fat loss is more commonly reported in women.

• Older people are more likely to report both fat gain and fat loss from the limbs, buttocks, and face. It may be that some of these changes are, in fact, natural changes which occur with ageing.

• The extent of immune recovery after starting anti-HIV treatments seems to predict the risk of body fat changes.

Avoiding body fat changes

Because the reasons for body fat changes in people taking anti-HIV drugs aren't properly understood, it's very hard to give clear advice about how to avoid them.

It used to be thought that the changes were only seen in people who took protease inhibitors, but in fact the changes are seen in people who have never taken this class of drug.

However, it is known that protease inhibitors can disturb the way the body handles fats and sugars.

There is some evidence that people who take d4T (stavudine, *Zerit*) are at greater risk of fat loss. It is also clear that people who start treatment with a combination that contains an NNRTI rather than a protease inhibitor are less likely to experience an increase in their blood fats and sugars.

Although you can delay the chances of developing lipodystrophy by not starting anti-HIV treatments, you need to balance this against the very real risk that you will become ill if you do not start anti-HIV drugs when you need them. Also, remember that fat loss seems to be more common amongst people who start anti-HIV treatments when their CD4 cell count is below 200.

Changing treatment to avoid body fat changes

There's no really strong evidence to show that changes from a protease inhibitor to an NNRTI will lead to an improvement in body fat changes. There is, however, evidence that this strategy might lead to an improvement in blood fats and sugars.

Changing from d4T to abacavir can lead to a very slow recovery of fat lost.

Stopping treatment because of body fat changes

Because changes in body shape can be very distressing, some people choose to stop their anti-HIV treatment completely because of them.

There's no evidence that this will lead to an improvement in body shape changes, although it might help to normalise levels of blood fats and blood sugars.

If you are considering stopping treatment because of body shape changes, it is important that you are aware of the risks that this could involve and that you talk to your doctor about regular monitoring. If you stop treatment:

• Your CD4 cell count is likely to fall back to its pre-treatment level within six months or less, regardless of how high it is when you stop. It will continue to fall.

• If you had an AIDS-defining illness before you started anti-HIV treatment, you are five times more likely to experience a decline in your CD4 cell count to back below 200 (the point at which you become vulnerable to other AIDS-defining illnesses).

• If you stop treatment with a CD4 cell count below 200 then you are at risk of developing an AIDS-defining illness immediately.

• If you are taking drugs such as 3TC (lamivudine, *Epivir*), nevirapine (*Viramune*) or efavirenz (*Sustiva*), which take a long time to clear out of the body, you run the risk of developing resistance during the withdrawal period. If you want to start treatment again with the same drug or drugs, it or they may no longer work.

• If you start treatment again, your blood fats and sugars are likely to return to their normal level.

Treating fat gain

There are currently no treatments to reverse fat gain. Some people who stopped treatment completely have reported small improvements. Although changes in diet and exercise will help improve your overall health, they are not effective against fat gains caused by anti-HIV drugs.

There are, however, a number of experimental treatments which are being used to treat fat gain. These include human growth hormone, anabolic steroids, and a diabetes drug called metformin. Because these drugs haven't been proven to be effective against fat gain caused by anti-HIV drugs, you may only be able to get access to them if you enroll in a clinical trial designed to assess how good they are when used in such a way. Ask your doctor if this is possible.

Surgery is being as explored as a remedy for fat gain at the back of the neck.

Treating fat loss

Fat loss from face, limbs and buttocks cannot be restored by any available treatment.

However, several forms of facial reconstructive surgery have been used to help remedy the appearance of fat loss from the face. The most promising of these is called *New Fill* (polylactic acid).

Studies from the UK and abroad have shown that *New Fill* can reverse the appearance of facial wasting and lead to an improvement in a person's quality of life, self-esteem, and confidence.

New Fill is administered by a course of injections into the cheeks, normally spaced over several weeks. The injections fill out the sunken area and encourage tissue growth.

It's not known for how long treatment with *New Fill* will remain effective. So far, it seems that a single course of injections will help to remedy the appearance of fat loss from the face in most people for two years. However, it may last longer in some people. On the other hand, there have been reports of some people needing much more frequent treatment.

The most commonly reported side-effect is soreness and swelling in the area where the injections are given. *New Fill* is safe to use with anti-HIV drugs.

Access to *New Fill* from the NHS is limited. However, it's hoped that as more evidence about its effectiveness emerges, this will change. Some, but not all, HIV clinics will provide free treatment to their patients. If you cannot get it for free, private treatment costs between £800-£1,200 per course.

Other cosmetic treatments for facial wasting that are being considered include fat transfer, collagen injections and hyaluronic acid.

Living with body shape changes

Body shape changes, in themselves, do not appear to be medically dangerous. However, they can cause physical discomfort and emotional problems. If you are becoming depressed because of changes in your body shape, make sure that you tell your doctor. Treatments for depression work well in people with HIV, and you might find a referral to see a counsellor or psychologist useful.

Changes in your metabolism

Anti-HIV drugs can also disrupt your metabolism – the way your body processes the things it needs to work properly.

Specifically, anti-HIV drugs can cause abnormal levels of blood lipids – cholesterol and triglycerides.

Cholesterol

There are two types of cholesterol. HDL cholesterol, often called good cholesterol, and LDL, or bad, cholesterol.

Levels of HDL cholesterol are often reduced in people with HIV and other chronic illnesses. High levels of LDL cholesterol indicate that you are at risk of heart disease, and increases of LDL cholesterol are often seen in people taking anti-HIV drugs.

If you have high LDL cholesterol, the following factors increase your risk of heart disease even further:

• Smoking.

• High blood pressure.

• A family history of heart disease.

• Being physically unfit.

• Age over 45 for men and age over 55 for women.

• Diabetes or insulin resistance.

• High blood sugars.

• Being very overweight, particularly with a lot of fat around the middle.

• Use of stimulant recreational drugs like cocaine or amphetamines.

It is particularly important to monitor LDL cholesterol levels if you are taking a protease inhibitor.

Triglycerides

Triglycerides are fatty acids derived from fat, sugar and starches in food. These travel through the bloodstream and are stored in tissues or in the liver.

Glucose

Glucose is a form of sugar found in the blood. High levels of glucose can increase the risk of heart disease.

Insulin

Insulin is the substance produced by the body to control glucose levels in the blood. Some people taking anti-HIV drugs need to produce more insulin to keep their blood levels of glucose normal. This is called insulin resistance. It may be necessary to have your insulin levels tested.

Symptoms of metabolic changes

Abnormal levels of fats and sugars in the blood can sometimes cause symptoms including:

• Tiredness.

• Dizziness (due to high blood pressure).

• Loss of concentration.

• More frequent urination.

• Thirst.

However, some people don't notice any symptoms, even when they've had abnormal levels of fats and sugars for a long time and are at risk of heart disease.

Heart disease and anti-HIV drugs

Levels of fats in your blood may start to rise when you start anti-HIV treatment, particularly if you are taking certain protease inhibitors. Sometimes they can increase so much that it's necessary to change your diet, start exercising, or take a medication to control them.

Large studies of people taking protease inhibitors have shown that they have a slight, but nevertheless significant, increase in their risk of heart disease.

If you have any existing risk factors for heart disease, your anti-HIV treatment should be carefully chosen to ensure that it doesn't raise your risk even further.

You should have your cholesterol, triglyceride and glucose levels monitored each time you have a routine clinic visit.

Looking after your heart

There is a lot you can do to help keep your blood lipids within safe limits. The information on diet, exercise, and stopping smoking in this book is a good place to start.

Lipid-lowering drugs. If you have high blood lipids, your doctor might prescribe lipid-lowering drugs. These are used to treat heart disease and hardening of the arteries. There are three classes of drugs available:

- Statins. This class of lipid-lowering drug has been used successfully in people with HIV. Statins are particularly effective at reducing levels of LDL cholesterol. Most statins can interact with protease inhibitors, but the drug pravastatin can be safely used with protease inhibitors. The main side-effect of statins is muscle weakness. Liver and kidney functions also need to be monitored.

- Fibrates. This class of drug lowers triglycerides and can also effectively lower LDL cholesterol. However, fibrates should not be taken if you have liver of kidney problems or if you are pregnant. On the other hand, fibrates seem less likely than statins to interact with protease inhibitors.

- Fish oil. A fish oil preparation that is rich in omega-3 fatty acids can reduce elevated triglycerides. However, you need to take a large number of pills every day for it to be effective. Fish oil can increase levels of HDL cholesterol.

Some drugs are also being investigated to see how effective they are at controlling glucose and insulin in HIV-positive people. These include metformin, sulphonylureas, and glitazones.

Peripheral neuropathy

Nerve damage can be a very painful side-effect of some anti-HIV drugs, and can also be directly caused by HIV itself.

Neuropathy is damage to the nerves. Nerves transmit signals within the brain and spinal cord (the central nervous system or CNS), and extend from the CNS to the muscles, skin and organs. The nerves that are outside the CNS are called the peripheral nervous system (PNS). They detect sensations, such as pain, and control movement.

Some of the peripheral nerves control body functions over which we have no conscious control, such as blood flow to the organs or the movement of food through the intestines. This is called the autonomic nervous system.

Symptoms

Peripheral neuropathy usually involves damage to the nerves in the feet or, less commonly, the hands. The symptoms can range from mild tingling and numbness through to excruciating pain that makes it impossible even to wear a pair of socks. Usually both sides of the body are affected equally.

Occasionally the autonomic nervous system can be affected, causing symptoms such as dizziness, diarrhoea and sexual dysfunction (inability to obtain or sustain an erection).

Neuropathy as a side-effect of anti-HIV drugs

Among people with HIV, neuropathy is commonly caused by certain medical treatments. It is a significant side-effect of several anti-HIV drugs – in particular, ddC (zalcitabine, *Hivid*), ddI (didanosine, *Videx*), d4T (stavudine, *Zerit*) and, to a lesser extent, 3TC (lamivudine, *Epivir*).

It can also be caused by other drugs prescribed for people with HIV, such as the antibiotics dapsone and intravenous pentamidine, the anti-TB drug isoniazid, and the anti-KS drugs vinblastine and vincristine.

If you take more than one of these drugs, the risk of developing neuropathy may be increased. If you have previously had neuropathy caused by something else, such as HIV itself, you may also be more likely to develop neuropathy from taking one or more of these drugs.

If you do develop drug-related neuropathy, it is important to stop taking the drug(s) promptly (but do try to get your doctor's advice before making any changes to your medical treatment). Once the drug has been stopped, the neuropathy may continue to get worse for a couple of weeks, but then it nearly always goes away over time. Later, you may be able to go back onto a reduced dose of the drug(s) without the neuropathy returning.

In the meantime, your doctor can prescribe treatments to reduce the pain, such as carbamazepine or amitriptyline. In severe cases, you may need strong painkillers. Trials have shown that a drug called L-Acetyl-Carnitine can help reduce the symptoms of neuropathy.

Other causes

There are several different causes of nerve damage among people with HIV.

Some causes are not linked to having HIV. For example, anyone who consumes large amounts of alcohol or certain recreational drugs like cocaine, heroin or speed can develop neuropathy; the best treatment is to stop or reduce your intake of these substances. Alcohol-induced neuropathy needs specific vitamin treatment from a doctor.

Neuropathy can also be caused by a shortage of vitamin B12, which can be relatively common among people with HIV. If medical tests confirm that you have a vitamin B12 deficiency, your doctor may offer supplements of vitamin B12 by injection (tablets are largely ineffective because vitamin B12 is poorly absorbed in the gut). Increasing the vitamin B12 content of your diet may also help a little; foods that are rich in the vitamin include fish, dairy products, kidneys, liver, eggs, beef and pork. Ask to see a dietitian at your clinic for more advice.

Some infections can cause neuropathy directly, such as cytomegalovirus (CMV) or HIV itself. These cases are best treated by tackling the underlying cause, such as using anti-CMV drugs or anti-HIV drugs, respectively.

Further reading

NAM factsheets, *Blood pressure, Blood problems, Cholesterol, Diarrhoea, Facial wasting, Fatigue, Lactic acidosis, Lipodystrophy, Nausea and vomiting, Neuropathy, Pain* and *Stroke.*

Anti-HIV drugs, HIV therapy, and *Lipodystrophy,* booklets in the information for HIV-positive people series produced by NAM.

'Anti-HIV therapy' in NAM's *HIV and AIDS Treatments Directory.*

Why don't I feel better?, leaflet produced by the Terrence Higgins Trust.

New life, *New Fill,* by Edwin

I had almost died in 2001, but thanks to an eight-drug salvage regimen I came back to life. Still my body and face bore the scars of lipodystrophy: thinning legs and bum, evidenced by varicose veins in my shins; central fat gain, evidenced by the increasingly larger jeans and baggier T-shirts I needed to hide my growing belly; and then, finally, deep lines in sunken cheeks and the shape of my skull obvious at my temples. I started seriously working out at the gym and changed my diet, gaining muscle where some of the fat used to be in my thighs, bum, and arms, and I soon lost much of my central fat accumulation. But my face remained lined and I felt that I had lost my looks – something that, as a vain gay man, bothered me more than I care to admit. And as an eight-year relationship came to end in the winter of 2001, I felt that I was now destined to live this hard-gained new life alone.

I found myself not being able to look at photographs of myself that showed me smiling, since the lines in my face deepened. In fact, as I stood in front the mirror pulling back the skin on my cheeks to see what my face had looked like before, I made a decision to try and smile less in general.

At first, I turned down an offer of *New Fill* from my Brighton HIV doc, saying that there must be much worse cases of facial wasting than mine. But after meeting an acquaintance who had had the treatment, and was glowing with confidence, I found the guts to ask for *New Fill* and in February 2003, I had my first appointment with Dr Gillian Dean – Brighton's *New Fill*-experienced doctor.

The treatment was not pain-free, but not as bad as root canal treatment at the dentist. But after the treatment was over, I was led into a small room and left alone with a mirror. It didn't really register at first that it was I who looked back at myself. Then I noticed how full my cheeks looked –almost too full, actually. Had I turned into a chipmunk? Was this Dr Dean's first disaster? I turned away and looked back again, this time more admiringly. Yes, the wasting was gone, but as Dr Dean explained when I subtly mentioned how full my cheeks looked, the effect at first is the bulk of liquid that contains *New Fill*. After a while, the liquid becomes absorbed and what is left is a thickening of the skin: that is why it takes three or four *New Fill* treatments to reach the required thickness.

That night, I looked at myself for a long time and realised that what the *New Fill* had done was not just fill my face and erase what I considered to be battle scars inappropriate to the way I wanted to live my life today, but also give me back the self-confidence that the lipodystrophy had imperceptibly eroded.

Chris's peripheral neuropathy

My peripheral neuropathy was caused by d4T, or was it ddI? I forget, it's such a long time ago.

The peripheral neuropathy I've experienced is different from that caused by HIV. The pain I've experienced sears through my big toes and top of my feet like hot cinders. It's transitory, passing in barely a second.

It doesn't sound like much, and goes unnoticed by people around me. Not surprising, as it normally just causes an involuntary twitch of the foot or leg.

My pain affects both big toes, and both feet, usually at the same time. It shoots across my instep and up into my calf muscles. There's no way of predicting when the pain will occur or how long it will last for.

The problem's not just the experience of the pain. It's what it does to me. It saps my will to live. I wilt, I lose my ability to concentrate, I'm overcome by a desire to collapse into sleep. This can last for a whole day – a whole day I'll never have again.

There are other physical symptoms as well. But these are more an expression of the emotional pain that peripheral neuropathy causes me. The pain forces a moan from my throat, my eyes smart with a deep searing wetness. Like the twitch in my leg or foot, all this goes unnoticed by the world around me.

People try to be helpful. A concerned friend recommended ibuprofen. "It's not that kind of pain," I reply. I don't think she understood.

What Michael did about his peripheral neuropathy

I took anti-HIV drugs in the belief that they would make me better. And true enough, within weeks of starting them my viral load fell back to undetectable and my CD4 cell count started a steady rise, banishing the minor illnesses which were plaguing my everyday life.

Well, something else started to plague my everyday life, and that was peripheral neuropathy. Quite simply it was the worst pain I've ever been in, and no painkiller, over-the-counter or prescription, seemed to make the slightest bit of difference.

To start with, I was reluctant to admit I had a problem. My test results were just so good. I didn't want to do anything which might give HIV a chance again. However, the pain became so bad that after a month of suffering I told my doctor how much pain I was in.

Without a moment's hesitation he recommended a treatment change. There were, he stressed, other drugs available, and there was no need to for me to suffer.

I still had my doubts. Both the drugs offered to me as alternatives – AZT and abacavir – seemed to have their own problems. However, my pain was such that eventually I opted for abacavir.

My viral load remained undetectable and my CD4 count continued to rise, and my peripheral neuropathy started to heal – very, very slowly. However, even though it's now years since I changed treatment I still have numbness and occasional pain in my feet. I've learnt that there's nothing to be gained from toughing through side-effects and that if you can do something about them, you should do it.

Symptoms and illnesses

Symptoms

It's worth knowing the range of symptoms you might experience so you can seek medical advice as soon as possible when you need it.

People with HIV get all the routine illnesses such as colds and flu that HIV-negative people get. So a chesty cough or diarrhoea could just be the result of the latest bug doing the rounds. But it could be something more serious, particularly if you have a low CD4 cell count. If your symptoms last for more than a few days, then you should see your doctor as quickly as possible.

What's more, anti-HIV drugs can cause side-effects. On the whole, these are minor and go away with time, but they can be more serious, and in certain circumstances dangerous.

Being able to get medical advice in an emergency is important. So it's worth finding out how you can get help from your clinic in an emergency or outside normal opening hours. You should also make sure that you are registered with a GP, who are the only doctors who can visit you in your home in the event of an emergency.

Doctors will always begin by asking you about your symptoms and examining you for signs of infection or allergy. They may then do a range of tests. Your doctor should explain what these tests are and why they are being undertaken.

Fevers and tiredness

These are sometimes called 'constitutional' symptoms because they affect the whole of the body. They can be the result of your body's attempt to fight an infection, and so can be caused by many different illnesses, and can also be caused by allergic reactions to some medicines.

Taking paracemtamol can help reduce fevers, but should be used with caution by people with liver problems.

Night sweats

These are a common problem, and may be either mild and infrequent or quite severe, resulting in the need to change your bed linen or clothes.

Causes

If it is a new problem and accompanied by a fever, an acute infection is often the cause. More specific causes include tuberculosis and lymphoma. If the night sweats are intermittent and/or localised, then HIV infection is usually responsible; this is inconvenient but not a significant medical concern. Anxiety can also result in night sweats.

What to do

It is important to try to track down any infections (other than HIV itself) that could be causing the sweats, especially if they are accompanied by fever. Practical measures such as taking an aspirin or paracetamol before sleeping may be helpful. If severe and accompanied by other symptoms of HIV disease, then anti-HIV drug treatments may be considered.

Chest and breathing problems

Chest problems are very common and can be can caused by colds, flu, smoking, asthma, and bronchitis. However, people with HIV are particularly vulnerable to some potentially life-threatening chest infections, such as PCP pneumonia and tuberculosis. Coughs and difficulty breathing should be taken seriously, particularly if the symptoms last more than a few days. It's also worth knowing that breathing problems can be a symptom of a severe allergic reaction to certain medicines.

Standard tests used if you have chest or breathing problems include:

- Checking your temperature. A high temperature can be a sign that you have an infection, and if your temperature goes above 102, you should see your doctor as soon as possible.

- A blood count. A blood sample is taken to see if your red blood cells, which carry oxygen, are depleted.

- A chest x-ray. This will show if there is inflammation or fluid on the lungs.

- A sputum culture. A sample of spit or phlegm is taken to see if there is any sign of infection.

In some circumstances, you may need to have a bronchoscopy. This involves passing a very small tube down with a tiny camera attached down a nostril or the throat into the lungs. A small tissue sample, called a biopsy, may also be taken. Bronchoscopies are only performed if doctors are uncertain what the cause of a chest problem is. They can be uncomfortable and if you need to have one you will normally be offered *Valium*.

Skin problems

Skin problems are common in people with HIV.

A common skin complaint in people with HIV is seborrhoeic dermatitis. This can cause scaly patches on the skin, and can be successfully treated with ointments.

A red rash might be the result of an allergic reaction to a medicine. If this happens to you, see your doctor as soon as possible.

Small, painful blisters around the mouth, genitals and anus can be caused by herpes simplex virus. Herpes can be controlled using aciclovir (for more information see *Sex and HIV*).

Small colourless bumps on the skin with a pearly top can indicate that you have molluscum contagiosum (molluscum for short). You are particularly likely to get this if you have a low CD4 cell count, and they can spread around the body quite rapidly. They are treated by freezing them off or by surgery. If you develop them before starting anti-HIV treatment you may well find that they go away by themselves once your immune system strengthens.

Small cauliflower-like growths are probably warts. For more information see *Sex and HIV*.

Black, purple or dark brown spots on the skin can be a sign of the AIDS-defining cancer Kaposi's sarcoma. To have this properly diagnosed, a sample of skin from the affected area needs to be biopsied. KS has become quite rare since effective anti-HIV treatments became available, but it can still be quite serious, so if you notice any unusual marks on your skin, make sure you bring them to your doctor's attention.

Mouth problems

Good dental hygiene including twice-daily brushing and flossing once a day will help you avoid most routine mouth problems.

However, people with HIV, particularly those with a low CD4 cell count, can be vulnerable to oral thrush, a fungal infection. Keep an eye out for white patches in the mouth. These can be painful, particularly if they are at the top of the throat, and can also cause an unpleasant taste. Oral thrush is easy to treat with a single dose of anti-fungal medication or lozenges. Once you start taking anti-HIV treatment and your immune system gets stronger, you'll probably find that you stop getting thrush.

If the white patches in your mouth are slightly hairy, then you might have an infection called oral hairy leukoplakia. This is caused by a virus and is treated with aciclovir. Again, you're likely to stop getting it once your immune system gets better after starting anti-HIV treatment.

Herpes blisters can affect the lips and mouth and can be treated with aciclovir. Mouth ulcers are more common in people with HIV, particularly people with lowish CD4 cell counts, but mouthwashes can help relieve the pain they cause. Mouth ulcers can also be a side-effect of some anti-HIV drugs.

Digestion problems

Pain or difficulty swallowing can be caused by oesophageal problems. The oesophagus is the tube that food passes down. Pain in the abdomen, nausea, vomiting, diarrhoea and constipation can all indicate stomach problems.

If these problems last more than a few days, or you start to lose weight, then see your doctor. Also, remember that most anti-HIV drugs can cause digestive problems, but these tend to pass with time and drugs can be taken to help control the symptoms.

Eye problems

You should have a periodic eye test, just like everybody else, to check your vision.

If you have a very low CD4 cell count, you should take problems with your vision very seriously. Blurred vision, blind spots, eye pain, or spots moving across the eye can all be symptoms of CMV (cytomegalovirus). This can be treated, but treatments work best if any eye damage is caught early.

Head problems

Everybody gets headaches from time to time. However, some anti-HIV drugs can cause problems with the head, as can certain infections, if you have a low CD4 cell count.

If you have any problems with your head lasting more than a few days, or any headaches which don't go away with normal painkillers such as paracetamol or ibuprofen, then see your doctor.

Side-effects caused by anti-HIV drugs tend to go away after time, and if they don't and you find that the head problems you are experiencing lower your quality of life, then speak to your doctor. It may be possible to change your medication.

Brain infections, such as toxoplasmosis and meningitis, are rare since the introduction of effective anti-HIV treatment. So too is AIDS-related dementia and lymphoma involving the brain. But if you experience symptoms of confusion, memory loss, poor concentration, speech problems or blackout tell your doctor immediately, particularly if you have a low CD4 cell count.

Depression is more common amongst people with HIV. For more information see *Mental health*.

Nerve problems

People with HIV can also experience problems with their peripheral nerves. This is called peripheral neuropathy, and it can be caused by HIV infection itself, or be a side-effect of drugs used to treat HIV and some other infections.

There is a lot more information on peripheral neuropathy earlier in this chapter.

Illnesses

The following is a summary of some of the more common illnesses that people with HIV can get. The list is not comprehensive, and it's worth remembering that the success of anti-HIV treatments means that many of the illness listed below are now very rarely seen in people with HIV in this country.

However, the pneumonia PCP and tuberculosis both affect about 200 people a year in the UK. Cases of these illnesses often occur in people who are unaware that they are HIV-positive.

Treatments are constantly improving, so only very basic information about treatments has been included. More comprehensive information can be found on NAM's website www.aidsmap.com.

Most illnesses are caused by one of the following:

- A virus. These are simple organisms which reproduce using the building blocks of your own cells. This makes it very hard to get rid of them.

- Bacteria. These are single-cell organisms that antibiotics can kill.

- Protozoa and parasites. These are more complex organisms.

- Fungi. Yeasts and organic growths.

- Cancer. Cancers develop when your own cells develop out of control.

However, it's possible that you have already been infected with the organisms which cause many of the illnesses listed in this section. This is because they are very common across the population and only cause problems if the immune system is damaged and unable to keep them in control. Even then, there are sometimes effective treatments to stop the illnesses flaring up (preventative treatment or prophylaxis).

Candidiasis (thrush)

This is a fungus that can affect wet and warm surfaces, such as the mouth, throat, vagina, anus and top of the penis. It looks a bit like cottage cheese and can be painful. Treatments vary depending on its severity, and are effective. Thrush can begin to appear before your CD4 cell count falls below 200.

CMV (cytomegalovirus)

Cytomegalovirus means great cell virus. It can affect the eyes, gut, lungs and nervous system. If not treated early, it can cause very serious problems such as blindness. CMV occurs in people with very advanced HIV disease.

Treatment for CMV used to be given by intravenous injection, but more recently effective oral treatments have become available.

Cryptococcal meningitis

Cryptococcus is a fungus found in bird excrement. In humans, it usually infects the lungs, causing a chest infection, but can rapidly infect the meninges (the lining of the brain) causing fever, headache, stiff neck and confusion. A lumbar puncture is needed to properly diagnose it. Meningitis occurs in people with very advanced HIV disease.

Different treatments are used depending on the severity of the infection, and in very severe cases these drugs can have quite severe side-effects. After recovering from meningitis, it is important to take prophylactic treatment to stop it coming back.

Cryptosporidiosis

Cryptosporidiosis, normally abbreviated to just crypto, is caused by a parasite that gets into the gut. It is normally transmitted in the water supply, or by contact with human or animal excrement. It causes watery diarrhoea, which can lead to very rapid weight loss. It can also infect the liver, causing inflammation.

Crypto often clears up by itself after a few weeks in people with less damaged immune systems. Although many drugs can be used to treat it, none are completely effective. Anti-diarrhoea and rehydration treatments are important in limiting the severity of the illness. It is also wise to see a dietitian if you get crypto, to make sure that you are getting enough nutrients from your diet.

HIV encephalopathy

This disease, sometimes called AIDS dementia complex or HIV-associated dementia, is caused by HIV's direct effects on the central nervous system. The first symptoms consist of minor changes in behaviour, coordination and concentration. Sometimes, those affected become apathetic or withdrawn. In some cases, it becomes much worse, resulting in a loss of control of movement, schizophrenia and suicidal impulses.

Many other illnesses can cause nervous or mental health problems, and HIV-associated dementia is very rare. However, it can occur in people who have very low CD4 cell counts.

The only effective treatment is anti-HIV therapy, and the success of anti-HIV treatments is the main reason why HIV-associated dementia is now so rare.

Kaposi's sarcoma (KS)

KS is a cancer which occurs most commonly on the skin, but can also affect the organs and intestines. It is thought to be caused by a type of herpes virus that is sexually transmitted. Most cases of KS in this country have been seen in gay men.

KS looks like purple, brown or black marks on the skin. These can look like bruises, bites or other infections, so a biopsy of the affected area is needed to confirm KS.

KS normally develops when you have a low CD4 cell count. The best way of treating it is to boost the immune system. Anti-HIV treatment regimens based on either protease inhibitors or NNRTIs have been shown to be equally effective at getting rid of KS. Individual lesions on the skin can be frozen off, and KS affecting the internal organs or intestines can be treated with chemotherapy or radiotherapy.

Lymphoma

This is cancer of the lymphatic system: the body's internal drainage system. It is normally seen in the lymph nodes, which swell up, but it can spread throughout the body. Symptoms include night sweats and fevers, but remember that many infections can cause these symptoms, as well as swelling of the lymph nodes.

Lymphoma has become a lot less common since effective anti-HIV treatments became available, and when it does develop, it can often be successfully treated with chemotherapy or radiotherapy.

MAI

This is caused by a bacteria similar to tuberculosis. It can be caught from soil or tap water. It only affects people with very severely damaged immune systems, when it can cause weight loss,

fever and diarrhoea. If you have a very low CD4 cell count, you doctor might recommend that you take preventative treatment stop you getting MAI. There are a number of treatments agains MAI, but their success varies. As with many AIDS-defining illnesses, the best treatment is often to strengthen the immune system using anti-HIV treatments.

PCP (pneumocystis carinii pneumonia)

PCP and tuberculosis are the two most common AIDS-defining illness in the UK. PCP affects about 200 people every year. It is fungus that lives in the lungs and causes inflammation in a perso who has a damaged immune system.

PCP can be a very dangerous infection if not treated early, so you should always tell your doctor if you have a persistent dry cough and shortness of breath. Other symptoms include fever and night sweats.

There are highly effective treatments against PCP, the most common being co-trimoxazole, but this can cause an allergic reaction. To avoid this, your doctor may desensitise you to the drug by giving you a progressively larger dose each day, over a number of days.

PCP rarely develops in people whose CD4 cell counts are above 200, the point at which you should start taking anti-HIV treatment. If your CD4 cell count is below or around 200 you should take PCP prophylaxis, even if you are taking anti-HIV treatments, until your CD4 cell count increases. PCP prophylaxis also protects against toxoplasmosis (see below).

Thrombocytopenia

This means that you have a low number of platelets in your blood – small cells that help your blood to clot. It can cause bruising and, in serious cases, internal bleeding.

As it is often caused by HIV itself, the most effective treatment is HIV therapy. It is very important not to take anti-inflammatory

drugs such as ibuprofen, as they can make the condition worse and cause internal bleeding.

Toxoplasmosis

Toxoplasmosis, or 'toxo' for short, is caused by a parasite transmitted in raw or undercooked meat. Cat faeces is also a theoretical risk.

Toxo can cause cysts to form on the brain, leading to headaches, fever, drowsiness, and fits. Without treatment, these can become very severe and lead to coma.

The drug used to treated PCP, co-trimoxazole, is also effective against toxo – so the condition is very rare, partly because people who are at risk of toxo are already taking co-trimoxazole to stop them getting PCP.

Tuberculosis (TB)

TB and PCP are the two most common AIDS-defining illness seen in the UK, with around 200 cases of TB diagnosed in HIV-positive individuals each year. Worldwide, TB is the leading cause of illness and death in people with HIV.

TB is caused by a very small bacterium. It is a very serious infection and causes fever, coughing, chest pain and weight loss. Unlike nearly every other AIDS-defining illness, you can become ill with TB even when you have a relatively high CD4 cell count.

TB is treated with a combination of antibitotics, which are normally taken for six months. These have to be taken very rigorously, or you run the risk of developing multi-drug-resistant TB.

For more information on TB, you can read the free NAM booklet *HIV and TB*, which is available from HIV clinics or can be downloaded from www.aidsmap.com.

Illnesses in the age of anti-HIV treatment – cancers

Anti-HIV treatments have brought longer and healthier lives for many people with HIV. Indeed, side-effects of treatment are the most likely cause of ill-health in HIV-positive people now, and in many cases these either lessen with time or can be controlled.

However, around 500 people a year in the UK develop an AIDS-defining illness, and around 400 people die every year because of HIV-related causes. Although illnesses such as PCP and TB still cause illness and even death in people with HIV, it seems that cancers and coinfection with hepatitis B and/or hepatitis C are becoming more common as causes of illness and death in people with HIV.

Kaposi's sarcoma and non-Hodgkin's lymphoma have become rarer since the introduction of effective anti-HIV treatment, but still cause illness and death in people with HIV. Often, these people have very weak immune systems, but there have been cases of these cancers developing in people who are taking HIV treatments and have good CD4 cell counts.

Other cancers that are not regarded as AIDS-defining conditions appear to have become more common in HIV-positive people since effective anti-HIV treatment became available. There is no evidence that anti-HIV drugs cause these cancers. The increased rates of some cancers seen in people with HIV since the introduction of HIV treatment have come about because people are living longer, and not dying of other illnesses.

Anal cancer

Anal cancer is emerging as a health concern, particularly for HIV-positive gay men. Human papilloma virus (HPV), the cause of genital and anal warts, is the underlying cause of anal cancer, and anti-HIV drugs are not effective against HPV. There has been a very slight increase in the amount of anal cancer seen in people with HIV since the introduction of anti-HIV treatments. Doctors think that this could be because HIV-positive people are living longer.

Before cancer develops, pre-cancerous lesions, called AIN (anal intraepithelial neoplasia), form. These are graded AIN I, AIN II, and AIN III according to severity. It takes a long time for AIN to progress to anal cancer. In some cases, AIN may be removed surgically.

Anal cancer is treated aggressively, with a combination of chemotherapy and radiotherapy. Sometimes, surgery is also needed, and the overall cure rate is about 60%.

Some HIV clinics are looking at the value of screening people with HPV in their anus or rectum for AIN. This involves using a test very similar to the PAP smear used to detect pre-cancerous cervical cells in women. Although these tests aren't 100% accurate, the earlier AIN is detected, the greater the chance of effective treatment.

Lung cancer

People with HIV seem to be at increased risk of developing lung cancer. It's very rare, however, and the outcome is no worse in people with HIV than it is in those without HIV. In one study, all the HIV-positive people who developed lung cancer were smokers.

Testicular cancer

There's some evidence to suggest that testicular cancer is more common in HIV-positive men. The reason for this isn't known. Treatment works just as well in HIV-positive men as in HIV-negative men, and if you notice a lump in your testicles you should see a doctor as soon as possible. The sooner treatment is provided the better.

Cervical cancer

Since the mid-1990s, cervical cancer has been an AIDS-defining condition. Doctors have noticed an increase in the incidence of cervical cancer since effective HIV treatment became available.

It's important for HIV-positive women to have regular PAP smears.

Liver cancer

For information on liver cancer, see the section on *Illnesses in the age of anti-HIV treatment – hepatitis.*

Illnesses in the age of anti-HIV treatment – hepatitis

Increasingly, coinfection with hepatitis B virus or/and hepatitis C virus is becoming a cause of illness in people with HIV. Both these viruses affect the liver , can make you very ill and can be fatal.

Hepatitis B

Hepatitis B virus (often known as HBV) is an infection that can cause severe or even fatal damage to the liver. Long-term infection with hepatitis B can cause liver cancer, and rates of liver cancer in people with HIV are elevated because of hepatitis B and hepatitis C. Hepatitis B is quite common in some of the communities affected by HIV in the UK, as it can be contracted in the same ways as HIV, particularly through contact with blood, semen or vaginal fluid, and from mother-to-baby.

You should be tested soon after your diagnosis for hepatitis B, to see if you have been infected with the virus and are a carrier. A vaccine is available to protect you against hepatitis B. If you are uninfected, and a test shows that you do not have natural immunity against it, you should be vaccinated.

If you are coinfected with hepatitis B, doctors will regularly monitor your liver function using blood tests. Ultrasound examinations may also be performed, particularly if your liver shows signs of damage. In some cases, it may be necessary to perform a liver biopsy. This involves taking a small sample of tissue from the liver, under anaesthetic, for examination under a microscope.

Treatments are available for hepatitis B, and three drugs have been licensed. These are alpha-interferon, the anti-HIV drug 3TC (lamivudine) and adefovir (*Hepsera*). Tenfovir (*Viread*) and FTC (emtricitabine, *Emtriva*) are also effective against hepatitis B, but have not yet been formally licensed for the treatment of HIV/hepatitis B coinfection.

Having hepatitis B is not thought to make HIV progress faster. Anti-HIV drugs can be used safely and effectively in people with hepatitis B. However, when some people start anti-HIV treatment, they experience a short-term flare-up of hepatitis B. This is because the immune system is getting stronger and is fighting hepatitis B. Some doctors try to stop these flare-ups happening by starting treatment for HIV and hepatitis B at the same time. Some anti-HIV drugs can cause abnormal liver function, including ritonavir, indinavir, nevirapine, AZT and ddI and should be used with caution if you have hepatitis B.

British treatment guidelines recommend that if you have hepatitis B and HIV, your anti-HIV treatment should include a drug that is effective against hepatitis B. These are 3TC, tenofovir and FTC. Some doctors think that a combination including 3TC and tenofovir is a very effective treatment for both hepatitis B and HIV.

Because of the risk of developing drug resistance, you should only take anti-HIV drugs to treat hepatitis B as part of an anti-HIV treatment regimen. If you are going to take treatment just for hepatitis B (and not for HIV), you should take alpha interferon or adefovir.

Hepatitis C

Hepatitis C is transmitted through blood, and the sharing of injecting equipment is the most common route of hepatitis C transmission in the UK.

Many people also contracted hepatitis C before blood screening procedures and sterilisation were introduced, and 95% of people with haemophilia and HIV in the UK are also coinfected with hepatitis C.

The sexual transmission of hepatitis C is a controversial subject. It used to be thought that this was very rare. However, there have been recent reports of increasing numbers of gay men testing positive for hepatitis C. Many of these men are HIV-positive and their only risk activity was unprotected anal sex. Sexual activity that carries a risk of contact with blood, such as fisting, seems to have a particular risk of hepatitis C transmission.

Mother-to-baby transmission of hepatitis C is thought to be uncommon, but the risk is increased if the mother is also HIV-positive. A high hepatitis C viral load also increases the risk that a mother will pass on hepatitis C to her baby, and, as with HIV, a caesarean delivery reduces the risk.

Very few people experience symptoms when they are first infected with hepatitis C. When they do occur, symptoms include jaundice, diarrhoea, and feeling sick. In the longer term, about 50% of people with hepatitis C will experience some symptoms. The most common ones are feeling generally unwell, extreme tiredness, weight loss, depression, and intolerance of fatty food and alcohol.

Although a small proportion of people infected with hepatitis C clear the infection naturally, about 85% will go on to develop chronic hepatitis C. About a third of people will develop severe liver disease within 15 to 25 years.

The severity of disease can be affected by the strain of hepatitis C you are infected with. Men, people who drink alcohol, people who are infected with hepatitis C when they are already into middle age, and people with HIV seem to experience faster hepatitis C disease progression.

Hepatitis C can cause liver fibrosis and cirrhosis. This damages the liver to such an extent that it cannot work properly, causing jaundice, internal bleeding, and swelling of the abdomen. Chronic infection with hepatitis C can cause liver cancer. Liver cancer is especially likely to happen in people with cirrhosis, particularly if they drink heavily.

There's also some evidence that smoking can speed up the rate of cirrhosis and increase the risk of liver cancer.

Liver cancer is difficult to treat, and often surgery is the only option. Small tumours can be removed, but there's a high chance of them recurring. Chemotherapy is not effective against liver cancer.

You should be tested soon after your diagnosis with HIV to see if you are also infected with hepatitis C. Unlike hepatitis B, there is no vaccine against hepatitis C, and if you are in a group at high risk of infection with hepatitis C, it's recommended that you should have frequent tests to see if you have been infected.

A test is also available to measure hepatitis C viral load (PCR). Unlike the HIV viral load test, this is not an indicator of when to start treatment. However, it is used to show how effective treatment for hepatitis C is and how long it should continue for.

Liver function tests can give an indication of the extent to which hepatitis C has damaged your liver. Liver ultrasounds and liver biopsies may also be used.

It seems that people coinfected with HIV and hepatitis C are more likely to develop liver disease than people who are only infected with hepatitis C. However, hepatitis C does not seem to increase your risk of becoming ill due to HIV, developing or dying of AIDS, or responding less well to anti-HIV treatment.

Anti-HIV treatment can be used safely and effectively if you are coinfected with HIV and hepatitis C. However, you may be at greater risk of experiencing the liver side-effects which some anti-HIV drugs can cause, and you and your doctor should have this mind when selecting which anti-HIV drugs to take. It also seems to be the case that people coinfected with HIV and hepatitis C are at greater risk of developing some of the metabolic disorders which anti-HIV drugs can cause (particularly insulin resistance and diabetes).

Drugs are available for the treatment of hepatitis C and you should receive your treatment and care from doctors who are expert in the treatment of both HIV and hepatitis C. This may mean that as well as seeing an HIV doctor, you may also need to see a specialist liver doctor.

Before you start treatment for hepatitis C, it is important to know which strain, or genotype, of hepatitis C you have been infected with, as this can predict your response to treatment and the amount of time you will need to take treatment for. There are several hepatitis C genotypes. Type 1 is most common in the UK, and unfortunately responds least well to the currently available treatments for hepatitis C.

Unlike anti-HIV treatment, treatment for hepatitis C is not lifelong. It consists of 24 or 48 weeks of treatment, and the length of treatment you receive will depend on the hepatitis C genotype you are infected with. A test after 12 weeks of treatment can predict if you are going to respond to treatment.

There are currently three drugs available for the treatment of hepatitis C. These are alpha interferon, pegylated interferon, and ribavirin. Treatment with a combination of pegylated interferon and ribavirin is becoming the standard treatment, as it produces better results and is the standard of care recommended by British HIV doctors.

If you have a CD4 cell count above 200, then the aim of hepatitis C treatment is to eradicate infection with hepatitis C completely. Although over 50% of people who are only infected with hepatitis C achieve this, the response rate is much lower in people with HIV.

Other aims of treatment include normalising liver function, reducing liver inflammation and reducing further damage to the liver. If you are ill because of HIV, then the aim of hepatitis C treatment is likely to focus on improving your tolerance of anti-HIV drugs, reducing the risk of death from liver problems and improving your overall quality of life.

Hepatitis C treatment can have very unpleasant side-effects, including temperature, joint pain, weight loss, nausea and vomiting and depression. Other side-effects include disturbances in blood chemistry.

If you are taking ribavirin you should not take ddI (didanosine, *Videx*), d4T (stavudine, *Zerit*) or tenofovir (*Viread*), because of the risk of very serious side-effects, including pancreatitis and lactic acidosis. Nor should ribavirin and AZT (zidovudine, *Retrovir*) be taken together, because of the risk of anaemia.

The infection which is the greatest risk to your health should be treated first. If you have a good CD4 cell count and are not ill because of HIV, then you should be given the chance to start hepatitis C treatment before starting HIV drugs. However, if your CD4 cell count is below 200, or is rapidly falling, or you are ill because of HIV, then you should start HIV treatment first.

Liver transplants

An increasing number of liver transplants are being performed on people with HIV who are coinfected with hepatitis B or C.

You are most likely to be considered for a liver transplant if HIV hasn't done too much damage to your immune system, or you have responded well to anti-HIV drugs, and have a good CD4 cell count and a low viral load.

Liver transplants seem to be just as successful in people coinfected with HIV and hepatitis B or C as in people who are just infected with either hepatitis B or C. Studies have found that HIV-positive people are just as likely as HIV-negative transplant recipients to be alive three years after receiving their new liver.

Organ transplant is a very specialist medical skill, and there's a chance that the hospital where you receive your HIV care may not be a centre with expertise in this area. This could mean that you are referred to another hospital.

If you have a successful liver transplant, you will need to take medication to stop your body rejecting your new liver for the rest of your life. You'll still have to take your anti-HIV medication as well.

Further reading

NAM factsheets: *Blood problems, Dementia, Diarrhoea, Fatigue, Genital warts, Hepatitis B, Hepatitis C, Immunisations, Kaposi's sarcoma, Liver, Mouth problems, Nausea and vomiting, Non-Hodgkin's lymphoma, Pain, PCP, Skin problems, Sight problems* and *Tuberculosis.*

HIV and hepatitis, HIV and sex and *HIV and TB,* booklets in the information for HIV-positive people series produced by NAM.

'Symptoms and illnesses' in NAM's *HIV and AIDS Treatments Directory.*

'HIV-hepatitis coinfection' in NAM's *AIDS Reference Manual.*

The risks of Hepatitis C, leaflet produced by the Terrence Higgins Trust.

TB – my experiences by Nick

This might sound odd, but I was really shocked when I became seriously ill because of HIV. I was even more shocked when it turned out to be tuberculosis.

I was diagnosed with HIV in the early 1990s. At that time, there was only one drug – AZT – and I was sure that HIV would kill me within about ten years. Well, by the summer of 1994 nothing had happened. My CD4 cell count was just as high as the day I was diagnosed and, to be honest, I felt healthier than ever. It really felt like a kind of phony war – the regular clinic visits for tests were nothing more than a minor inconvenience, and I even dared to think that I might be one of the handful of individuals I'd read about who remained healthy with HIV for years on end.

With these thoughts in mind, I didn't pay too much attention to a newspaper report I read about the first increase in tuberculosis cases in the UK since vaccination, effective antibiotics, and improved housing and nutrition came along after the last war. I wasn't even concerned when I read that many of the cases involved people with HIV. I also felt reassured because I'd had a tuberculosis vaccine as a teenager. And on top of it all, I just felt so healthy.

How wrong I was.

The first symptom was a mild, dull pain in my lower right chest. I felt certain it was just a pulled muscle and carried on as normal. I wasn't alarmed when I started waking up in the middle of the right with a light sweat on my forehead. It was summer, after all. And I also found an easy explanation, simple tiredness, for the severe breathlessness I experienced on my 16-mile Sunday run.

It was, however, much harder to explain away the temperature of 104 degrees I awoke with the following Monday. That something was seriously the matter was confirmed at the hospital by a chest x-ray showing a mass of fluid on my right lung – exactly where the pain had been for the past few months. Initially, I was treated for bacterial pneumonia. PCP pneumonia was ruled out as my CD4 cell count was about 500. I didn't get any better. Further tests over the next few days, which involved draining over two litres of fluid from my lung and a biopsy, confirmed that I had tuberculosis.

How could I have got tuberculosis, I asked myself. The answer was simple, I was HIV-positive and even the very mild immune damage I'd experienced was enough to undermine whatever protection my childhood vaccination offered and leave me vulnerable to infection with tuberculosis and the development of disease.

I was physically and emotionally wrecked. In the space of a fortnight, I lost a stone in weight and became very weak. I had to rely on my partner and friends to undertake household tasks for me. But just as severe was the emotional impact. The combination of anti-tuberculosis drugs quickly controlled my symptoms and, as I was careful to take every dose of my six-month course of treatment, I was completely cured. Although my CD4 cell count fell by about a half to 250, within six months I was able to run just as often and as far as before, with only the very occasional twinge of pain in my chest to remind me of the scarring caused by the tuberculosis.

But the emotional impact was much more permanent. I realised just how serious HIV was, and accepted for the first time that I'd probably have a series of severe illness over the coming years before a premature and inevitable death. As I result, I left work and planned as pleasant as possible a retirement for my last few years of life.

It hasn't quite worked out like that, thanks to the anti-HIV drugs I've been taking since 1998. But in summer 1994, effective anti-HIV treatments, and the hope that they've brought for me, were a very long way away.

Living with HIV and hepatitis C coinfection and haemophilia – Paul

For most people, coping with HIV is enough of a problem in itself, but when you throw in a lifetime disorder such as haemophilia, and then add hepatitis C virus to the list, it does complicate things.

I was born with haemophilia, so it's something I have known all my life, and something that I have grown up coping with. I've never known anything different. The damage to my joints caused by internal bleeding has left me with chronic arthritis, which impairs my mobility and causes daily pain.

I was diagnosed as HTLV-3 positive, as HIV was known, in 1985, and given little hope of a future, along with over 1200 others with haemophilia in the UK. There was no pre- or post-test counselling offered and very little advice. The only thing I was told for certain was that I wouldn't have long to live.

In 1992, I was told I had also become hepatitis C virus positive, through the same route of infection as my HIV – contaminated Factor VIII, the treatment I took to prevent internal bleeding.

I was told that HIV would cause my death many years before hepatitis C would be a problem and advised not to worry about it.

By 1998 I had numerous HIV-related illnesses, a very low CD4 count and an extremely worrying increasing viral load. I started antiretroviral therapy, which was a turning point for me, not only in addressing my HIV, but also in contemplating the effects of my other conditions.

Protease inhibitors have been shown to cause increased internal bleeding in people with haemophilia, so they were not an option. I was also concerned about the effects any drugs would have on my liver and the impact they may have on my hepatitis C. My hardest task at the time was finding information about co-infection. The HIV organisations knew about HIV and the Hepatitis organisations about hepatitis but neither seemed to know much about both viruses in combination.

I started treatment with a regimen of nevirapine and *Combivir*, which have luckily worked well – I am still on the same regimen six years later. However, four months into this medication, alarm bells were ringing about nevirapine and hepatic failure. My liver function test results had escalated since I began HIV treatment and I was in turmoil, worried that although one set of drugs were working well against the HIV, they might be causing increased hepatic problems. Again I struggled to find information, running back and forth between two hospitals and three different consultants – who never met each other.

Eventually, my liver function test results reduced. They were still abnormally high, but were now at a level that wasn't scaring me, or my doctors, too much.

The HIV drugs were working, and for the first time in 15 years I actually thought I might have a future. The advent of pegylated interferon and ribavarin gave me hope for treating my hepatitis C. I wanted to start treatment and agreed with my doctors to start a trial. I had weighed up the consequences, read as much as I could about what to expect and talked to other people who had undergone hepatitis C treatment. I discussed with my hepatologist and my HIV consultant, as well as both sets of pharmacists, what options were available and what possible HAART regimen changes could be made if needed.

I told most of my family and friends that I was to start hepatitis C treatment and planned my life so that I had time to cope with side-effects. By the time the trial was due to start, the hospital ethics committee had decided to exclude people with HIV. This was a devastating blow at the time, and didn't help my relationships with my doctors. The same hospital that had infected me with both viruses wouldn't give me the opportunity to try and treat one because of the other.

I heard many stories about the horrific side-effects that some people were having on this medication and by the time pegylated interferon was licenced, I had my reservations about trying treatment. By now I had more questions. I have hepatitis C-genotype one, which is the hardest to treat, needing twelve months' of therapy and still giving the poorest results. I knew that AZT and ribavarin were causing problems for the majority, and now I was scared about changing my HIV treatment regimen because it was working so well for my HIV. I didn't want to jeopardise the success of my HIV therapy, to have twelve months of hell and only a 25% chance of success if I endured the treatment. It all seemed too much of a gamble.

All my illnesses concern me. My arthritis hurts daily, I have to inject factor 8 when needed, my twice-daily visit to my pill box reminds me, as do the nausea and the night sweats, of my HIV – and my liver throbs at times. I don't know what the future holds, but I am hoping that hepatitis C medication improves before my liver deteriorates. It's a big gamble, but the last 20 years have also been a gamble, against all odds. I have been crossing my fingers and trying to stay informed along the way, and I will continue to do so.

The luxury of hypochondriacs, by Caroline Guinness

That anxious look I get from loved ones is very hard to take, and all I want to do is reassure them that everything will be all right. Complicated, isn't it?!

When I was first diagnosed with HIV, I felt very isolated. I had a gay friend with AIDS but I did not tell him about my diagnosis as I didn't want to worry him. He was very ill at the time and I felt my health was OK – the last thing I wanted to do was give him something else to cope with, so I looked after him and forgot about my own HIV.

The few friends I told at the time were shocked and very concerned about my health. Again, I did not want to worry them, so I did not discuss what I was going through. I became aware that I could no longer whinge about any aches, pains, colds or any other 'normal, everyday maladies', because to them it represented something far more serious.

I coped for a while by just being in complete denial, but I began to feel isolated and longed to be able to speak freely about my situation, longed to meet other women in the same situation as myself.

I met other positive women for the first time at a support group. It made an enormous difference, the relief of being able to talk, knowing they were feeling the same things, made me feel 'normal' for the first time in ages. I went on to run support groups and discovered, again and again, that no matter what the cultural differences might be, we all had basically the same problems – the main one being how to cope with our HIV status.

Then I started to realise that my (HIV-negative) friends were treating me differently. I had always offered a shoulder to any one of them who needed it. But what I began to find was that even if I could see that they were going through a difficult time, they did not seem to want to talk to me about it. Over dinner one night, a good girlfriend, having consumed rather too much alcohol, informed me that she did not feel she could confide her problems to me as she felt mine were so much bigger than hers...BINGO...I understood what was going on.

I tried tell my friends that their problems were relevant and of course I still wanted to be confided in and asked for friendly advice. Whenever I said this, I was always greeted with `but I don't want to worry you'. Luckily, as the years have gone by they have become used to my HIV, and our relationships carry on as normal. I never did want to be treated differently. Having said that though, I have learned to never complain about any illness unless I know it is really serious... and even then I play it down.

My circle of HIV-positive friends grew and I felt I had a great balance. Every now and then, I would meet up with my peers, have a few drinks and be able to talk about anything related to our status.

Since moving to the country, I have had little contact with my HIV-positive friends. One night last week I met up with a group of friends, one of whom was positive. It felt like manna from heaven, and without realising it, he and I immediately fell into 'HIV speak' and forgot about everyone else at the table – we could talk about our 'aches and pains' and not worry each other.

I think when you are suffering from a life-threatening illness you do not want to tell people about your everyday symptoms. I have realised that it is a luxury for healthy people to complain about their health. The usual advice to them is along the lines of: "Oh don't worry, it is only a cold/flu, everyone's going down with it, have some Lemsip, you'll be fine." The only people who seem able to say this to me are others in the same situation... who are also HIV-positive.

So to any healthy hypochondriacs reading this, do not feel guilty, you have a luxury I really miss. To moan and not be taken seriously... yes, please.

This first appeared in issue 87 of Positive Nation, February 2003. Many thanks to both Caroline and Positive Nation for giving permission to reprint it.

Daily health issues

Day-to-day hygiene

Generally, hygiene precautions for people with HIV need not be different from those for anyone else. This is because most of the opportunistic infections associated with HIV are not ones you `catch' from the environment. For instance, people with HIV are no more or less vulnerable to the common cold than anyone else.

A few simple basic hygiene guidelines make good sense:

• Wash your hands with thoroughly with soap and hot running water after using the toilet, handling rubbish or pet waste, and before and after preparing food.

• Wear strong rubber gloves and use very hot water and strong disinfectants when cleaning up anything messy such as diarrhoea, pet droppings and manure, or when gardening or dealing with rubbish.

• Make sure you use different cleaning cloths for kitchen surfaces and floors and the bathroom.

• If you have cuts on your skin, wash well under running water, encourage a bit of bleeding to flush out any germs, clean the cut with antiseptic and put a waterproof plaster over it.

• Get medical attention if you have a deep cut.

• Do not share toothbrushes or razors.

• Carefully dispose of sharp objects.

There are some other circumstances where it is worth taking extra precautions. Avoid children with chicken pox if you have never been exposed to it before. It is caused by the herpes zoster virus, which may cause shingles in HIV-positive adults.

Pets and animals

Some doctors warn that diseases such as toxoplasmosis, which can have very serious health implications for people whose immune systems are damaged, could be acquired from cats, birds or dogs. Others would agree that though this is true in theory, in practice, if you have owned your pet for a while, there may be no extra risk to you. This is because of the nature of opportunistic infections. Most of them involve the activation or reactivation of micro-organisms which entered the body in the past. On that basis, if you have had a particular pet for a while, you are unlikely to be at risk of catching anything new from it.

There is also evidence to suggest that the risk of acquiring such infections from animals is, in reality, low. One study has reported that people with HIV who owned cats were no more likely to develop toxoplasmosis during their illness than those who did not own cats. Changing cat litter on a daily basis will reduce the risk of toxoplasmosis. Clean the litter tray using rubber gloves, hot water and strong disinfectants.

Cats can also harbour the bacterial infection *Bartonella* (also known as `cat scratch' disease). Try not to let your cat lick open cuts, and try to ensure that it doesn't get fleas, as all of these can transmit *Bartonella*. Always wash your hands between touching pets and handling food.

Exposure to potentially harmful organisms can also occur when working with animals or gardening. For example, cleaning chicken coops or cleaning up pigeon droppings could expose HIV-positive people to infections, as could gardening without gloves.

If your job could lead to you coming into contact with potentially dangerous infections, then you should discuss this with your doctor and the occupational health department at your work.

Drinking water

On the whole, it's safe for people with HIV to drink water from the tap in the UK.

But if you have a severely damaged immune system, a little more caution might be needed. Water companies cannot guarantee that water supplies are free from *cryptosporidium* or other similar organisms which cause diarrhoea in HIV-positive people who have very low CD4 cell counts. Once contracted, *cryptosporidium* seems impossible to eliminate in HIV-positive people who have CD4 counts below 200 and leads to serious diarrhoea and inability to absorb food or fluids. It is a serious opportunistic infection, against which current treatments are only partially successful.

People who have CD4 cell counts above 200 appear to have developed enough immune response to control cryptosporidiosis, although they may experience some diarrhoea.

There were several outbreaks of cryptosporidiosis in London and Oxfordshire in the early 1990s, which caused severe diarrhoea even in HIV-negative people. These outbreaks have been traced to the water supply.

Thames Water, which provides water in London, says that it is impossible to filter drinking water for the *cryptosporidium* egg because the infectious dose is so low. Hundreds of gallons of water would need to be screened to find one egg. Unlike bacterial infections, which are able to establish themselves only when tens of thousands of bacteria get into the gut, ten *cryptosporidium* eggs are enough to cause severe diarrhoea.

If you fit your own filter against *cryptosporidium*, it should have a very fine mesh.

Filtered water should be kept in the fridge. If it is left at room temperature, it may actually be more vulnerable to bacterial contamination than plain tap water because filtering removes the chlorine which is added to water supplies. The main drawback of filtered water is the cost; over £100 for the filter and fitting.

The only other way to eliminate the organism is to boil drinking water for at least one minute. Such a lengthy boiling period is necessary in order to ensure that all the water has reached boiling point; an automatic kettle switches off when the water in contact with the filament has reached boiling point. Some experts on water safety say that this is not long enough to ensure the elimination of some organisms.

Many people assume that bottled mineral water is always safe, but this is definitely not true. Bottled water sources cannot be screened for *cryptosporidium* either, and other bacteria not present in chlorinated tap water have been found in some brands of bottled water.

It is important to remember that drinking water includes the water with which you brush your teeth and prepare or wash food (for people with CD4 counts below 200, this means being careful all the time). Drinking water also includes ice in drinks, which is made from tap water.

Drinking water may also contain other diarrhoea-causing bacteria. These have been isolated in bottled water as well as tap water, and the only way to remove these bacteria is either to boil water or to use a very fine mesh filter, even finer than the filters recommended for *cryptosporidium*. Jug filters, which are very popular, tend to remove chemical impurities but may not always screen out bacteria.

To make life easier, it may help to boil up water once a day and keep it in the fridge to use later on. Don't use boiled water that is over twelve hours old, even if it has been kept in the fridge.

Unfortunately, it is not always possible to monitor the quality of water which you drink or which is used in the preparation of food outside the home. In these circumstances, the best policy may be to avoid salads and other raw foods, and to drink bottled water from deep mountain springs, which are least likely to be contaminated with *cryptosporidium*.

Beer, pasteurised fruit juice and bottled/canned soft drinks do not carry the risk of *cryptosporidium* infection, but it's unknown whether wine could carry the infection.

Water outside the UK can present problems. Even in other European countries it is best to stick to boiled water or, if this is difficult, bottled water that comes from deep mountain springs. In tropical and subtropical countries, water presents a very serious health hazard to HIV-positive people. A large number of gut infections are water-borne, including some which cause life-threatening diarrhoea, and any traveller who returns from these countries with diarrhoea will tell you that, however tempting it may look, roadside food and drink is not worth the risk.

Swimming in the sea or in rivers may also be inadvisable for people with compromised immune systems, especially off the British coast. Several recent reports have highlighted extensive problems with water-borne infections contracted from polluted or sewage-ridden water. This is also known to be a problem in many Mediterranean resorts and a cautious approach would be to swim only in chlorinated swimming pools.

Food poisoning

If you have a strong immune system, your risk of getting food poisoning is no greater than it is for an HIV-negative person.

However, food poisoning can be a lot more severe in people with AIDS. It makes sense for everyone who has a low CD4 count to take extra precautions.

Salmonella is a definite risk for people with HIV. *Salmonella* is as much a problem in Britain as it is in other parts of the world. Another possible risk is listeria, another infection spread by food, which may cause particular problems for children with HIV. *Shigella* and *campylobacter* can also cause problems. Infections with these organisms can be hard to get rid of, and they can fail to respond to treatments which are effective in HIV-negative people.

Salmonella frequently infects chickens. This means that it is especially important to make sure chicken is cooked through, so that no red blood can be seen at all. Take special care with frozen chicken. Meat should be thawed in the fridge, not at room temperature. Wash your hands after handling uncooked poultry and make sure uncooked meat and poultry is not stored uncovered in the fridge near cold meats or dairy products. Ideally, wash eggs before cracking them, and cook them thoroughly until both the yolk and the white set. Do not use cracked eggs.

It is also advisable to avoid unpasteurised dairy products, including unpasturised milk, `live' yoghurt and some soft cheeses, which may also contain *salmonella* and listeria. Some people have advocated live yoghurt as a treatment for thrush. Although there is some evidence that this does indeed have benefits, it is important that people with HIV are aware that it may also carry some risk.

It may also be sensible to avoid farm animals and their droppings, since these can harbour infections such as *cryptosporidium*. Organically grown vegetables are often grown in a medium that includes raw manure, so it is wise to brush off as much dirt as possible and then clean the vegetables with boiled water.

If reheating or microwaving food, take care to ensure that it is properly cooked all the way through. Wash fruit and vegetables properly, and keep cutting and preparation surfaces clean. When on holiday in warm climates, the risk of food poisoning may well extend to salads and fruit. Food which you know has been immediately and thoroughly cooked is safest. Do not use food after its sell-by date.

International travel

Going to a foreign country can be daunting, as even straightforward everyday tasks may suddenly require learning a whole new set of steps. Just the strain of daily life can become stressful. In addition, you are likely to be exposed to new and potentially dangerous bugs for which your immune system will be unprepared. It is wise to have a check-up at your clinic before you go, and to ask about any extra precautions you need to take. If you are currently using any medications, ensure that you take an adequate supply with you, as they may be hard or impossible to obtain abroad. Medicines should be clearly labelled, and, at some countries' customs and immigration points, it will help to have a doctor's letter stating that you need the treatments. There's a lot more information on travelling with your medication in the chapter *Travel*.

It is sensible to research local medical facilities before travelling to another country, particularly if local medical care is likely to be relatively poor.

Make sure that you have the right travel and medical insurance. Most policies won't cover medical conditions that you know were aware of when you took out the policy. For more on travel insurance, see the chapter *Travel*.

Coughs are a common problem among travellers, and you may be at particular risk during air travel, when large numbers of people are confined in a small space, breathing recirculated air.

Travellers' diarrhoea is usually caused by the contamination of food or water with faecal bacteria by people who have not washed their hands. It affects about 40% of travellers to developing countries, even when they have perfectly intact immune systems, and can be a particular problem for people with HIV. The most common cause of diarrhoea after travelling is giardiasis, which can be treated quite easily in people with HIV.

Vaccinations and immunisations

An immunisation (often called a vaccination) is designed to protect the recipient against an infectious disease. People with HIV should receive the vaccinations against hepatitis A virus and hepatitis B virus. It's not recommended that people with HIV receive live vaccines such as the BCG tuberculosis jab, as this might cause illness.

Sex

There are good reasons why you should still consider having safer sex even if you are HIV-positive.

First of all, you might infect somebody else with HIV. In England, there have been cases of men being sent to prison for infecting their sexual partners with HIV, and a man has also been imprisoned in Scotland for this.

Then there's the issue of sexually transmitted infections, which at the very least can be unpleasant and inconvenient, and can also make it more likely that you can pass on HIV during sex. If left untreated, some sexually transmitted infections can cause serious health problems, particularly if your immune system is very weak.

There is some evidence that unsafe sex might damage the health of people with HIV and several cases of reinfection or superinfection with drug-resistant strains of HIV have now been presented.

In the early 1990s, an American study involving thousands of HIV-positive gay men found that men who had unprotected anal sex experienced faster disease progression and became ill with HIV-related illnesses faster than those who said they only had safer sex. A study involving Kenyan sex workers showed that women who had unprotected sex had more sexually transmitted infections and lower CD4 cell counts.

For more information see the chapter *Sex and HIV*.

Reinfection/superinfection

Although it is clearly established that drug-resistant HIV can be transmitted to previously uninfected people, it is less clear if it can be transmitted to people already infected with HIV. There have, however, been several case reports from around the world of HIV-positive people being reinfected with another strain of HIV after having unprotected sex – and doing less well on their HIV treatment as a consequence.

It seems that reinfection is, however, rare, and in a number of the reported cases the individuals were taking a break from their HIV treatment when they became reinfected

This is quite a controversial subject. It is being looked at very closely by doctors around the world, and more information is being published on it all the time.

Different strains of HIV

Many different strains of HIV exist, some of which are more aggressive than others in the test-tube. It has been suggested that transmission of an aggressive strain (to an individual who is already infected with a less aggressive strain) may trigger the onset of AIDS.

This might happen because the aggressive strain could overwhelm the immune system. For instance, a person's immune system may have responded quite successfully to initial HIV infection, so that the dominant strain of HIV in the body is one which is less harmful to the host. Reinfection with another strain could tip this balance: the host's immune system may be unable to contain a new, more aggressive virus strain, which could therefore be able to replicate rapidly. The aggressive new virus could soon overtake the strain already present, and become the dominant strain. Another theory is that the new strains might selectively infect certain types of cells or tissues which had been largely unaffected previously, and so lead to faster disease progression.

It has certainly been demonstrated that people have been infected with two different sub-types of HIV, but no one is sure when those infections might have occurred. Some researchers have suggested that infection with a second strain of HIV is most likely to occur in the first few months of primary infection, because this is the time when the immune response against HIV is least strong. Others argue that the immune response may not be protective, and that re-infection could occur at a later stage.

Co-factors

Although there are these doubts about the importance of re-infection with HIV, there are reasons to believe that other virus infections and sexually transmitted infections may speed up disease progression.

In the first place, many infections are likely to cause HIV to reproduce simply because they stimulate the immune system. That immune response will include the activation of latent HIV in immune cells, leading to the production of new HIV and the infection of further cells.

For instance, after being infected with cytomegalovirus (CMV), people with HIV infection have been shown to suffer increases in HIV replication. But CMV and some other viruses can also assist HIV in the infection of new cells, and speed up HIV replication in cells which are infected with both HIV and CMV. The same goes for other herpes viruses, Epstein-Barr virus (which causes glandular fever) and hepatitis B virus. All these viruses have the potential to provide `keys' to cells which HIV would otherwise be unable to infect. Almost all of these viruses are transmitted through sexual or body fluid contact.

Sexually transmitted infections

For most people with HIV, standard treatments for sexually transmitted infections work just as well as they do in HIV-negative people.

However, if your immune system is very weak, you might need a longer course of antibiotics to treat infections such as gonorrohea and syphilis.

Viral sexually transmitted infections can also be more serious and harder to treat if you have HIV. For example, people with HIV may be at greater risk of having more frequent and more painful attacks of genital herpes.

In people with HIV, it can also be harder for the immune system to clear infection with HPV, the virus that causes genital and anal warts. Some strains of this virus can cause cervical and anal cancer, and even after the introduction of anti-HIV treatments, doctors have seen an increase in the incidence of these cancers in people with HIV.

Hepatitis B virus is also sexually transmittable and people with HIV are recommended to be vaccinated against it. There's evidence that hepatitis C virus can also be sexually transmitted.

Oral-anal contact, or rimming, can lead to gut infections.

It is up to each individual to decide what sex practices they want to keep up, which they want to modify, and which they want to stop. For instance, one might still make the choice not to use condoms for penetrative sex with a regular HIV-positive partner. At the other end of the spectrum, one might decide to begin to use condoms for oral sex.

Recreational drug use

Nearly every person with HIV uses some form of drug. Most people use legal drugs like coffee, tea or chocolate, and many others drink alcohol or smoke tobacco. A large number of people with HIV also use illegal drugs.

In this section, information is provided on alcohol, tobacco and so-called recreational drugs.

Drugs and the law

For the very latest information on the adverse effects and legal status of drugs, you might want to look at the website of the UK drugs information charity Drugscope, www.drugscope.org.uk.

Generally, drugs in the UK are controlled by two laws: the Medicines Act and the Misuse of Drugs Act. The Medicines Act bans the non-medical use of some licensed pharmaceuticals. The Misuse of Drugs Act is concerned with the use of banned drugs, which are placed into different categories. Offences involving Class A drugs carry the stiffest penalties, and offences involving Class C drugs the lightest. A first offence involving possession of drugs is likely to involve a fine or caution. But this would mean that you have a criminal record. Regular offenders, and people who sell or smuggle drugs, can expect to face a prison sentence, and having HIV is unlikely to mean that the courts will deal with you more leniently.

Alcohol

Alcohol is a drug and comes in many forms, including beer, cider, wine, 'alcopops' and spirits such as whisky, gin and vodka.

Alcohol is legally available in the UK from licensed outlets to people aged over 18 years and is enjoyed and used safely by many people. However, alcohol is a major cause of health and social problems, and, after tobacco, causes more deaths in the UK than any other drug.

Alcohol relaxes the brain and body, and is normally drunk for its pleasant effects. Because of its power to alter mood and make physical changes, it can also lead to physical, psychological and social problems. Many people find that moderate drinking (a unit or two of alcohol per day) helps relieve stress, encourages relaxation and acts as an appetite stimulant. A unit of alcohol is equal to a half-pint of normal strength beer or lager, a pub measure of spirits, a glass of wine, or a small glass of sherry or port.

Health agencies recommend that men should not drink more than 3 to 4 units of alcohol per day. For women, the daily limit is 2 to 3 units. This advice applies regardless of whether you drink daily, weekly or somewhere in between. Drinking all your weekly limit in one session (often called binge drinking) can lead to poor coordination, vomiting, exaggerated emotional reactions (including sadness, tearfulness, anger and aggression) and can even unconsciousness. Women who are pregnant, or planning to become so, are advised to drink no more than 1 to 2 units per week.

A hangover the next day – headache, dry mouth, feeling sick and tired – is a very common consequence of heavy drinking the night before. These effects are caused by dehydration and toxicities, so if you drink alcohol, you should drink plenty of water as well.

As even small amounts of alcohol can have an effect on your coordination, reactions and judgments, you should never drink even small amounts of alcohol and then drive or operate machinery.

Extremely heavy drinking can lead to coma and even death.

Long-term heavy alcohol consumption (10 or more units a day in a man or 6 or more in a woman) can cause ill health, affecting the liver, heart and brain. Drinking every day can also lead to physical and psychological dependence on alcohol.

In addition, people who drink heavily often don't eat well and this can cause further health problems. Alcohol is a depressive drug and can cause or make worse mental, psychological or emotional problems. Used in conjunction with other drugs, such as over-the-counter pain-killers like paracetamol, alcohol can have more serious effects.

There is no evidence that moderate drinking (a unit or two of alcohol a day) does any harm to people with HIV. However, if you have hepatitis or high levels of blood fats, then you may have to cut down your alcohol consumption or stop drinking alcohol altogether.

Heavy drinking can affect your immune system and may slow down recovery from infections.

Heavy alcohol use can have potentially serious consequences for people taking anti-HIV drugs. Alcohol is processed by the liver and a healthy liver is necessary for the body to process medicines effectively. The blood fat increases caused by some anti-HIV drugs can be made worse by heavy drinking.

People who have hepatitis as well as HIV are advised not to drink alcohol at all, or to keep alcohol consumption to an absolute minimum.

People whose liver has been damaged by drinking too much alcohol (especially if they have hepatitis) are more likely to experience side-effects from anti-HIV drugs, particularly protease inhibitors.

Alcohol can react badly with certain medicines (for example some anti-TB drugs and some antibiotics) so it is a good idea to check with your pharmacist whether it is safe to drink alcohol with any new medicines you may be prescribed. However, there is no significant interaction between any of the currently available anti-HIV drugs and alcohol.

Alcohol can cause vomiting. If you vomit within an hour of taking a dose of your anti-HIV drugs, or any other medicine you have been told to take, then you should retake the dose.

If you are concerned about your drinking, speak to a member of your health care team, who will be able to direct you to somebody who can help. Alcohol Concern, one of the UK's largest alcohol charities, can be contacted via www.alcoholconcern.org.uk, or phone Drinkline on 0800 917 8282. More information on Scottish support services is online at www.alcohol-focus-scotland.org.uk, or phone 0141 576 6700.

Amphetamines (speed)
Also see the section on crystal meth below

Amphetamines are stimulants normally taken orally, although they can be dissolved in water, snorted, or injected. After cannabis, amphetamines are the most widely used illicit drug in the UK, and are classified as a Class B drug in the Misuse of Drugs Act, unless they are prepared for injection, when they are Class A.

Amphetamines cause the heart rate to increase, appetite to diminish, mood to improve, and the pupils to dilate. Users often report a 'rush' of confidence lasting three or four hours before they begin to 'come down'. Feelings of anxiety and agitation take over from this point. Repeated use of amphetamines can lead to tolerance of the drug, meaning that you have to take more to achieve a 'high'. Symptoms of anxiety, paranoia and panic can also set in. Prolonged and heavy use can lead to mental disturbances.

Amphetamine use postpones, but does not remove, the need to eat. Regular users often suffer from weight loss and malnutrition. This reduces the body's ability to fight infection, and this is a major concern for people with HIV.

There is no clear evidence that HIV-positive users of amphetamine experience faster disease progression, but see the section on crystal meth (methamphetamine).

Anabolic steroids

Anabolic steroids are hormones which are commonly used as drugs to build muscle mass. Body builders and, increasingly, regular gym users often use anabolic steroids in four-week cycles, to improve the effects of their training.

HIV-positive men are sometimes prescribed anabolic steroids or testosterone replacement therapy if they have low natural levels of testosterone or have lost a lot of lean muscle mass.

Steroids can be highly toxic to the liver, and can also cause acne, male pattern baldness, sexual problems and shrinking of the testicles. Women who use anabolic steroids can develop masculine characteristics.

Steroids bought at gyms are often counterfit or contaminated in some way and can be particularly toxic to the liver and cause nerve damage.

There is controversy about the effect of anabolic steroids on the immune system. Some researchers have argued that they are immunosuppressive, but a study looking at the immune systems of HIV-positive men given prescribed steroid treatment for wasting showed that they did not suppress the immune system. However, it is known that steroid use can increase levels of LDL (bad) cholesterol, so they should be used with extreme caution and under close medical supervision if you have raised blood fats due to your anti-HIV medication.

Needle-sharing by steroid users carries exactly the same risk of HIV transmission as needle-sharing for recreational drug use.

Barbiturates (downers)

Barbiturates are used medically, to calm people down and as sleeping pills. Barbiturates are a prescription-only drug and are classified as a Class B drug if they are used illicitly. Possession is not, however, a criminal offence.

Barbiturates affect the central nervous system, causing a clammy feeling, and depending on the dose, the effects last between three and six hours. They can cause clumsiness, happiness and mental confusion – and unhappiness can also be caused by barbiturates.

Large doses can cause unconsciousness, breathing problems and death. Death from overdose is a very real danger, as a dangerous dose is very close to a normal safe dose. The chances of overdose are increased if barbiturates are taken with alcohol. The risks of barbiturate use are increased if the drug is injected.

The body can rapidly become tolerant of barbiturates, leading to both physical and mental dependence. Withdrawal can involve symptoms of irritability, sleeplessness, sickness, twitching, convulsions and delirium.

Heavy users are more vulnerable to chest complaints and hypothermia.

Cannabis

The legal status of cannabis changed recently in the UK, when the drug was reclassified from Class B to Class C.

Cannabis can be smoked, usually with tobacco, eaten, drunk in a 'tea' or snorted as a snuff. The drug affects the central nervous system and, as a result, users may experience relief from pain, feel light-headed, relaxed or sleepy. The drug can also stimulate appetite; the so-called 'munchies'. However, cannabis is also known to impair co-ordination, and can cause nausea and vomiting as well as anxiety and paranoia, which, with long-term use, may become chronic.

Medicinal use of cannabis is illegal and therefore there is little verifiable evidence of the drug's effects when used in the management of chronic health conditions. However, cannabis is widely used illegally for medicinal reasons, often for the relief of pain or as an appetite stimulant. In 1996, a clinical trial in San Francisco found that people with HIV wasting disease who used cannabis were more likely to put on weight. The drug is also widely used to relieve insomnia and the symptoms of anxiety and stress. It is also used by people with multiple sclerosis as a muscle relaxant.

In recent years a small number of people have been prosecuted for growing and consuming cannabis for medicinal purposes. In most cases a suspended sentence has been issued, but recently a jury returned a not guilty verdict, and in another example a judge threw out the case.

The UK Government is currently reviewing the evidence on cannabis use. Cannabis extracts, called cannabinoids, are already legally used in licensed pharmaceuticals, mostly pain killers and muscle relaxants, but these can only be obtained on prescription. These products do not make users feel 'high' or have any of the other narcotic effects of cannabis.

Short-term risks of cannabis use include anxiety, panic, and paranoia. Memory and attention may also be affected, as might the ability to drive or operate machinery. Research suggests that cannabis use in teenagers is a predictor of later mental health problems. Use during pregnancy has been associated with low birth-weight babies.

If the drug is smoked, long-term use is known to cause many smoking-related respiratory and cardiovascular diseases such as asthma, bronchitis, emphysema and heart disease. This may be of particular concern to people with HIV who have suffered lung damage from TB, or to those with increased lipids from anti-HIV medication, as this may increase the risk of heart attack. There is also evidence that smoking cannabis can cause cancers of the mouth, throat and lungs.

Chronic loss of memory and shortened attention span have been observed in long-term users of the drug, in some cases even after their use has ceased, and there is evidence that long-term users can develop psychological dependency on the drug. In a recent survey, daily use of cannabis by teenagers was found to substantially increase the risk of developing depression later in life and the use of cannabis has also been linked with an increased risk of schizophrenia.

It is not known how cannabis reacts with anti-HIV drugs. A small American study found that cannabis use did not impact on the effectiveness of the protease inhibitor indinavir (*Crixivan*), even though the drugs use the same mechanism to pass through the body. Like any mood- or consciousness-altering drug, cannabis may have an impact on people's ability to adhere to their medication schedule. People planning to use cannabis, or any other recreational drug, may need to develop strategies to help them take their medication at the right time and in the right way.

Cocaine

Along with most other recreational drugs, government statistics suggest that more people are using cocaine (coke, charlie, snow, powder, marching powder) and the cocaine derivative, crack (freebase). In the UK, both cocaine and crack are illegal class A drugs. Dealing carries a maximum penalty of life imprisonment and unlimited fine, and possession can mean up to seven years in prison and a fine of £5,000.

Cocaine is a stimulant made from the leaves of the South American coca shrub. It comes in the form of a white powder, costing between £30 and £100 per gram. Usually snorted into the nose, it provides a feeling of excitement, exhilaration and self-confidence lasting for about 15-30 minutes. Cocaine can also be rubbed into the gums and into the anus or vagina before penetrative sex. Rarely, cocaine is also made into a solution for injection.

Crack is sold in the form of small rocks, which are smoked either in cigarettes or in a pipe. Historically, crack has been associated with poor urban populations, but is in fact used by people from a wide social spectrum.

Cocaine users may take many doses to maintain the high, which can cause anxiety, paranoia and a tolerance for the drug, meaning that larger doses have to be taken to achieve a similar high. Although not addictive in the same way as heroin or opiates, users can become psychologically dependent on the transient high which cocaine provides and find that they suffer anxiety, depression or severe tiredness if they stop using the drug.

Longer-term use of both cocaine and crack can cause severe anxiety, clinical depression, psychotic episodes, aggression, weight loss and malnutrition. Both drugs have also been shown to cause potentially fatal heart problems including heart attack, angina, irregular heart beat and inflammation and enlargement of the heart.

In common with most other street drugs, users are rarely sold a pure form of cocaine. The drug is often 'cut' with other cheaper drugs such as amphetamines (speed), talc or detergents, which can be poisonous or cause irritation, leading to infection.

Snorting cocaine can damage the membrane between the nostrils, leading to bleeding and eventual erosion. There have been reports that sharing snorting equipment may permit the transmission of hepatitis C virus. Rubbing cocaine into the gums, vagina, or anus can cause ulceration, which could increase transmission of HIV or other sexually transmitted infections. Sharing injecting equipment also presents a risk for transmission of HIV, hepatitis viruses and other blood-borne infections.

Cocaine is not metabolised by the body in the same way as anti-HIV drugs, so there does not appear to be cause for concern about interactions between them.

Test-tube studies suggest that cocaine alters the functioning of the immune system in several ways, making immune cells more vulnerable to HIV. Experiments conducted in HIV-infected mice bred in laboratories found that mice exposed to cocaine had far fewer CD4 cells than mice not given the drug. This suggests that HIV disease may progress faster in regular cocaine users.

However, studies looking at regular cocaine use and disease progression in gay men have produced conflicting results. One study found no association, whilst another found that weekly cocaine use was associated with a greater risk of death. Because drug use may be an indicator of other social issues which may have a negative effect on health – such as poor access to health care, or other health problems – these types of studies can be difficult to interpret.

As with all recreational drugs, it is also wise to consider how use could impact on adherence to your HIV treatments. If you are worried about your recreational drug use, then your doctor or health care team will be able to refer you to an appropriate source of support.

Crystal meth (methamphetamine)

Also know as crystal meth, ice, tina, krank, or yaba, methamphetamine is a synthetic form of amphetamine, a stimulant drug.

Crystal meth has been popular on the US gay scene for over a decade, and there have been some alarmist reports about its use amongst gay men in the UK and Europe. However, it is unclear just how widespread use of the drug, which is very expensive and difficult to obtain, actually is.

Like amphetamine, methamphetamine is a class B drug. Possession carries a maximum sentence of five years and/or a fine and dealing carries a prison sentence of 14 years and an unlimited fine. If methamphetamine is prepared for injection, then legal penalties are more severe.

Methamphetamine can be bought as a pill, as a powder to be snorted through the nose or injected, or in a crystal form – ice – which is smoked in a pipe.

Methamphetamine brings on a rapid feeling of exhilaration, a perceived sharpening of focus and heightened sexual desire.

Smoking crystals of methamphetamine causes a rise in body temperature, an increased heart rate and rapid breathing.

Paranoia, short-term memory loss, rages and mood swings have been recorded.

There is anecdotal evidence that use of methamphetamine can cause people to become ill because of HIV more rapidly, to take more time to recover from infections and to respond less well to anti-HIV treatments. However, some people believe that this has a lot to do with users of the drug not taking their anti-HIV and other medication properly.

Rapid fall in CD4 cell count has been observed in methamphetamine users. However, as many users of methamphetamine have difficulty sleeping because of the use of the use, or don't eat properly, there may be other lifestyle factors involved in the quicker disease progression noted in some users.

Psychological dependence on the drug has also been reported, although it does not seem to cause physical addiction.

Taking large amounts of the drug can cause convulsions, problems with blood circulation, inability to breath, coma and death. However, deaths have been reported in people who have taken only small doses.

In the US there have been concerns about a link between the use of methamaphetamine by gay men and unprotected sex, particularly when used in conjunction with drugs to treat erectile dysfunction, such as *Viagra* and *Cialis*.

There has been a case report of an interaction between methamphetamine and the protease inhibitor ritonavir (*Norvir*). Methamphetamine is metabolised by the body using the same mechanism as ritonavir. Doctors also believe that inhaling poppers may make the interaction worse.

The use of any drug can interfere with normal sleeping patterns, affect appetite and interrupt routines. Some people have found that this is particularly the case with methamphetamine. If you are using the drug, it makes sense to consider how it might affect issues such as adherence to your anti-HIV medication. The drug has also been linked with an increased likelihood of having unprotected sex, so plan how to manage this.

Ecstasy

Ecstasy (E, X) is an illegal class A drug. Dealing carries a maximum life prison sentence and unlimited fine, and possession up to seven years in prison and a £5,000 fine.

Ecstasy has both stimulant and hallucinogenic properties. Its active ingredient is a synthetic drug called MDMA. Originally used in psychotherapy, from the late 1970s it started to be used on the club scene due to its ability to reduce inhibitions, give an energy boost, induce relaxation and give intense pleasure by releasing the neurotransmitter serotonin.

The drug is sold in tablet form and, less frequently, as a powder. After about 30 to 45 minutes, the drug gives an intense 'high', which may last for several hours. Because the body becomes tolerant of the drug, people may end up taking larger quantities to induce similar feelings of euphoria.

Because ecstasy is illegal there have been no proper clinical trials looking at the risks of using the drug for people with HIV. The effects of ecstasy on the immune system and on HIV disease progression are therefore uncertain.

In 1996, a man who had recently started taking a combination of anti-HIV drugs, including the protease inhibitor ritonavir (*Norvir*), died after taking two and a half ecstasy tablets. An autopsy found that there was an unusually high amount of ecstasy in his blood, which may be partly explained by an interaction between the drug and ritonavir. Ritonavir boosts the amount of ecstasy in the bloodstream by between 200% and 300%, because the body uses the same process to break down both ritonavir and ecstasy.

Because other protease inhibitors (and NNRTIs and many other drugs) are metabolised using a similar process, there is a risk that ecstasy could interact dangerously with them, and there have been hospitalisations due to adverse reactions to ecstasy amongst people taking protease inhibitors.

If you've started a new treatment combination recently, the first four weeks, when your body gets used to the new drugs, are likely to be the riskiest time for interactions. Some doctors suggest that after this period, if you choose to take ecstasy, it may be safer to begin with a quarter or half a tablet first. This information is included here in order to help readers reduce risks, and has not been researched scientifically.

As with all recreational drugs, it is difficult to know what the ecstasy tablet you are using really contains. The doses found in street drugs are not controlled, and the ecstasy pill you buy might contain much larger quantities of the drug. Often, ecstasy will have been 'cut' with other substances which could be poisonous, or with other drugs, usually amphetamines or LSD, but occasionally heroin.

In the short-term, ecstasy can cause dehydration, headache, chills, eye twitching, jaw clenching, blurred vision, nausea and vomiting and, like many drugs taken to get 'high', is commonly accompanied by a 'come-down'.

People can have an allergic reaction to the drug, which can be fatal (though deaths related to ecstasy are very rare relative to the extent of its consumption). The drug has also been associated with heart and lung problems, dramatic increases in body temperature, kidney failure and liver damage. The potential liver toxicities of ecstasy and other recreational drugs are of particular concern to people with HIV, as liver damage can itself make you very ill as well as stopping the body from processing anti-HIV drugs properly.

Long-term use has been linked to poor mental health, depression, psychotic episodes and memory problems.

If you are using ecstasy or planning to do so, then think about discussing this with your doctor or another member of your health care team. Most are quite happy to discuss drug use and can provide helpful information on minimising risks.

As with all recreational drugs, it is wise to consider how use could impact on adherence to your HIV treatments or other areas of your health or life.

GHB

GHB (gammahydroxybutyrate) has recently become popular on the club scene, with users reporting an alcohol-like high with potent positive sexual effects. However, its possession and use recently became illegal after a series of deaths were associated with its use.

GHB affects the release of dopamine in the brain, causing effects ranging from relaxation to deep sleep, and coma. The drug also lowers blood pressure and can cause breathing difficulties.

A case has been reported in which levels of GHB were increased to life-threatening levels when taken along with a protease inhibitor. A man who was taking ritonavir and saquinavir became deeply unconscious after taking a half-teaspoon of GHB. Doctors believe that the ritonavir and saquinavir slowed down the metabolism of GHB and caused a near-fatal reaction.

Heroin
See opiates

Ketamine
Ketamine is an anaesthetic which makes people feel detached from their immediate environment.

Possession of Ketamine is not illegal. However, dealing the drug is illegal under the Medicines Act. It comes in a white powder which can be snorted, dissolved or injected. It normally takes effect after about 20 minutes. The body heats up and users have reported a range of different experiences including an altered sense of their body, hallucinations, difficulty moving or even completely freezing. This is often called a "K-hole", and involves difficulty communicating and even breathing and swallowing.

The effects of long-term ketamine use include memory loss and psychological disturbance. Several deaths have been reported due to the use of the drug in the UK. Although no specific interactions with anti-HIV medication have been reported, use of the drug could affect adherence to anti-HIV medication.

LSD

LSD (lysergic acid diethylamide, often known as acid) is a Class A drug. It is taken orally and normally begins to take effect after about 30 to 60 minutes. Its hallucinogenic effects last up to eight hours, although some people report "trips" lasting as long as 24 hours.

LSD is not thought to affect the immune system and no specific interactions with anti-HIV drugs have been reported. However, when "tripping" on acid adherence to anti-HIV medication might be difficult or even impossible.

Opiates

These include heroin and methadone and are made from the opium poppy. Heroin is a Class A drug. Methadone is controlled by the Medicines Act.

Opiates are normally injected, smoked or sniffed. They depress the nervous system and have a euphoric effect. Tolerance of opiates develops quickly, as does dependence.

Use of opiates can cause chest problems and constipation. Sharing the equipment used to inject opiates can lead to infection with tetanus, hepatitis B and C, HIV, and can cause blood poisoning and abscesses.

Use of opiates can lead to malnutrition and self-neglect.

Methadone is a form of opiate normally supplied on prescription to registered addicts as an alternative to injecting. It is usually taken as a liquid. To withdraw from opiate use, addicts can gradually reduce their dose of methadone over a long period of time.

Methadone interacts with anti-HIV drugs. The drug is known to increase levels of AZT (zidovudine, *Retrovir*) in the blood. Doctors are often very cautious about giving people taking methadone protease inhibitors and will often admit them to hospital for observation for a short time. The protease inhibitor nelfinavir (*Viracept*) reduces methadone levels. The NNRTIs have differing effects on methadone levels. Nevirapine (*Viramune*) increases levels of methadone, whereas efavirenz (*Sustiva*) reduces levels of methadone, particularly in the early stages of treatment.

There is conflicting evidence about the effect of using opiates on HIV disease progression, with some studies finding that heroin users progressed to AIDS and death faster, while others did not. Since the advent of anti-HIV treatments, some evidence has emerged that opiate users become resistant to their anti-HIV drugs faster, probably due to poor adherence.

Poppers

Poppers are a nitrite-based drug. Amyl nitrite is used medically to ease the chest pain caused by angina. The drug gets its name from the small glass capsules containing amyl nitrite for the treatment of angina which used to be 'popped' under the nose and inhaled. Amyl and butyl nitrite started to be used recreationally, and have been popular with gay men for many years. More recently, they have become popular with clubbers of all sexualities.

In the UK, poppers are sold in small bottles, which contain a liquid form of butyl nitrite. It is very rare for amyl nitrite to be used as poppers, as its sale is illegal without prescription under the Medicines Act. The legal status of butyl nitrite has been the subject of court cases in recent years. The sale of butyl nitrite poppers is legal, largely because they are sold as 'aromas' or 'room odourisers' rather than as a drug to be inhaled. The possession of poppers, in either amyl or butyl nitrite form, is legal.

When inhaled, poppers cause blood vessels to dilate, allowing more blood to reach the heart. They also cause blood to rush to the brain, speed up heartbeat and relax muscles, providing an intense high lasting a few minutes at most. The drug is widely used to intensify pleasure whilst dancing and having sex. Sniffing poppers relaxes the anal sphincter muscles, allowing anal sex to take place more easily. As poppers dilate blood vessels, many men find that they lose their erection when sniffing them.

After-effects of sniffing poppers may include headache, skin rashes, weakness, sinus pains and burns if the liquid comes into contact with the skin. Sniffing poppers can also cause nausea and vomiting. People with heart or lung problems are advised to avoid poppers, as they can cause breathing problems. In very rare cases, excessive sniffing of poppers can cause the lips and skin to take on a blue tinge. This can be accompanied by vomiting, and shock, and unconsciousness may follow. In extreme cases, deaths have been reported.

The long-term effects of poppers have been a matter of considerable controversy, particularly as it has been argued that their use caused AIDS and particularly Kaposi's sarcoma. However, this view is not supported by any scientific evidence and studies comparing the effects of poppers on HIV-negative and HIV-positive gay men found that only those with HIV suffered any immune damage or progressed to AIDS. However, some animal studies have shown that poppers can suppress immune responses and can have cancer-causing effects. These studies have been criticised because of the relatively large amounts of nitrites given to animals. Any long-term immune damage or cancer-causing effect in humans remains to be proven.

There are no documented interactions between drugs used to treat HIV and poppers. However, sniffing poppers after taking the anti-impotence drugs *Viagra* and *Cialis* can result in a potentially dangerous, even fatal, drop in blood pressure. The dangers from sniffing poppers after taking *Viagra* or *Cialis* are increased if you are also taking a protease inhibitor as part of your HIV treatments. Protease inhibitors cause the amount of *Viagra* or *Cialis* in the blood to increase, and for this reason it is recommended that people prescribed protease inhibitors take only half the normal dose of *Viagra* or *Cialis* and do not use poppers at the same time.

As with any drug, it may be wise to consider how using poppers affects your wider health and lifestyle, particularly if you are using poppers with other drugs or alcohol. Some people report that using poppers may act as a trigger for unprotected sex and, if this is the case for you, you may wish to have a strategy in place to help you manage this.

Sexual dysfunction drugs

Viagra (sidenafil citrate) and *Cialis* (tadalafil) are treatments for erectile dysfunction which have become increasingly popular as recreational drugs, particularly amongst gay men, many of whom use the drug to counteract the impotence side-effect of other recreational drugs such as ecstasy. Several studies have linked use of *Viagra* and *Cialis* with increases in the amount of unprotected sex gay men are having and increased rates of sexually transmitted infections. However, it is unclear if this is because the use of these drugs enables men to have more sexual partners or just increases the amount of sex they are having. It's also possible that men just add the use of anti-impotence drugs to their existing risk-taking repertoire.

The most common side-effect of these anti-impotence drugs is headache. Neither *Viagra* nor *Cialis* should be used in conjunction with poppers, as this could cause a potentially dangerous drop in blood pressure.

Protease inhibitors and NNRTIs are metabolised by the body using the same method as *Viagra* and *Cialis*, and this can mean that you get very high levels of anti-impotence drugs in your blood, increasing the chances and severity of side-effects. For this reason, you are recommended to reduce by half the standard dose of both *Viagra* and *Cialis* if you are taking either protease inhibitors or NNRTIs, and not to take more than a single standard dose of either of these impotence drugs in a 48-hour period.

Smoking

Tobacco is a legal and widely used drug. However, smoking is addictive and it is beyond any doubt that smoking can severely damage health and cause early death. HIV-positive smokers may be more likely to get certain AIDS-defining illnesses if they have a weak immune system, and be at increased risk of developing the metabolic side-effects caused by some anti-HIV drugs.

Smoking, in itself, does not make HIV infection worse. The rate at which HIV disease progresses, or at which CD4 cells are lost, is no greater in smokers than non-smokers. Anti-HIV medication is just as effective in smokers as non-smokers.

However, there is very good evidence that people with HIV who smoke are more likely to get certain infections and AIDS-defining illnesses, particularly those affecting the chest. It's known that smokers are approximately three times more likely than non-smokers to develop the AIDS-defining pneumonia PCP. Oral thrush, a common complaint in people with HIV, is also more common amongst smokers.

Emphysema, a smoking-related illness, occurs much more commonly in HIV-positive smokers than HIV-negative smokers.

It's well known that smoking increases the risk of heart disease, high blood pressure, and stroke. It's thought that having a long-term illness like HIV might increase the risk of heart disease. Further, some anti-HIV drugs can cause increases in blood fats, and this can contribute to cardiovascular illnesses. If you smoke and take anti-HIV drugs, then your risks might be increased even further.

It's well established that smoking increases the risk of lung cancer. Although relatively rare, lung cancer seems to occur more often in people with HIV, even if they are taking anti-HIV drugs and have a well-controlled viral load. In one study, all the HIV-positive people who developed lung cancer were smokers.

Stopping smoking (or not starting in the first place) will significantly reduce your risk of developing heart disease and other cardiovascular illnesses. You are most likely to stop smoking and stay stopped if you are motivated.

Individual or group therapy has been shown to help people to stop smoking, and your HIV treatment centre may have a therapy group for individuals who are stopping smoking.

Cigarettes are addictive because they contain nicotine. Many people find that nicotine replacement therapy can help reduce the craving for cigarettes and make quitting easier. Your doctor may be able to prescribe patches, gum, or lozenges which contain nicotine, and there is no evidence that these interact with anti-HIV drugs. You can buy all of them over the counter.

The antidepressant drug bupropion (*Zyban*) has been licensed to help people stop smoking. However, it interacts with anti-HIV drugs of both the protease inhibitor and NNRTI classes, leading to an increase in the amount of bupropion in the blood. Make sure you tell your HIV doctor if you are thinking about taking bupropion. The drug also causes side-effects, including dry mouth, insomnia, headaches, and fits.

Many people find that alternative therapies, such as acupuncture and hypnotherapy, help them stop smoking. Exercise can also be helpful.

Quit is a UK charity which provides help to people who want to stop smoking. Their telephone advice and support service – Quitline – can be reached on 0800 002200. Their website is www.quit.org.uk.

Safer drug use

The importance of safer injecting

HIV can be transmitted by sharing injecting equipment, including water, spoons, needles and syringes. Safer injecting will reduce the chances of you passing on HIV, reduce the chances of you picking up other blood-borne infections, protect you from dirty hits, and protect you from pain and injury when you inject.

Essentials of safer injecting

Get hold of new needles. Find out where there is a needle exchange that provides them free of charge. They will usually offer other services as well.

Always use new needles when you inject. Have a plan to make sure that you have new needles with you when you need them so you never end up sharing needles with others.

Learn how to clean needles. This can be important for situations when you cannot get new needles.

Where to get new needles

Getting free access to new needles differs according to where you live in the UK. Some areas have needle exchanges, others have mobile services, and others have a pharmacy-based service.

Needle exchanges

These are specialist projects set up primarily to exchange used needles and syringes for new ones. They usually offer more than simple needle exchange – sometimes this includes primary health care. Workers in needle exchanges are normally very friendly and non-judgmental.

Mobile or outreach schemes

These are not usually run from a fixed location. These schemes might move from one venue to another, or be housed in a van or bus that visits certain locations at set times, or even be a home delivery scheme.

Pharmacy-based schemes

In some areas, needle exchanges are operated through chemists. Some schemes require minimal registration details, although other are more informal. Even if there is no formal scheme, chemists may sell needles.

How to find needle exchanges

Your HIV clinic will be able to help you. Most needle exchange services will offer safer injecting advice, primary healthcare, safer sex advice, condoms and referrals to other specialist services.

Cleaning injecting equipment

It's best to have a new syringe and needle for every injection. If this is not possible, cleaning your injecting equipment will offer some protection against the transmission of HIV and other infections.

Bleach method

Fill a container with clean, cold water. Draw the water up the needle and fill the syringe, flush out the syringe away from the clean water and repeat. Then fill the container with household bleach, and repeat the cleaning process. Finally, repeat the process again with clean water.

This will kill HIV, provided the bleach is of sufficient strength. Thick bleach can be difficult to draw up a needle, and can also be difficult to flush out, so use thin bleach whenever possible.

Washing-up liquid method

Fill a container with clean, cold water. Draw the water up the needle and fill the syringe, flush out the syringe away from the clean water and repeat. Add a generous squirt of washing-up liquid into another container and dilute with cold water. Repeat the cleaning process, making sure you do not squirt the dirty water into the container with the washing-up liquid. Finally, clean with clean water, using the same process as described above.

Washing-up liquid can kill HIV, but again, thick washing-up liquid can be difficult to draw up fine needles, and bubbles can be left in injecting equipment bythis process, so it needs to be thoroughly flushed out before the equipment is used for injecting.

Boiling method

Boiling equipment for five minutes will kill HIV and other infections. However, most disposable syringes will melt if boiled.

Disposing of used injecting equipment

Your local drugs team will be able to tell you about the disposal facilities in your area. Never over-fill containers given to you to dispose of your injecting equipment – two-thirds full is the maximum. With larger syringes, you can put the needle into the barrel of the syringe and push the plunger in until it bends the needle. Put the used equipment in a bag and place in a bin. You can put smaller syringes and needles in a drinks can, crush the can, then put it in a bag and place in a bin.

Dealing with overdose
Reducing the risks of an overdose

The risks of overdosing can be reduced by:

• Being sure of the drug you are injecting.

• Being sure of the strength of the drug supply.

• Not returning to the same dose of a drug after a break, as your tolerance of this drug will have been reduced.

• Not injecting alone or in a place where you cannot be easily found.

• Taking a reduced dose of any new supply.

If you find someone who has taken an overdose

• Lie the person on their side with their airway clear – this will make sure that they don't choke on their own vomit or suffocate.

• Call an ambulance immediately.

Further reading

NAM factsheets, *Diarrhoea, Immunisations, Preventing infections*, and *Sleep*.

HIV and hepatitis, HIV and sex and *Nutrition*, booklets in the information for HIV-positive people series produced by NAM.

'A healthy lifestyle' in NAM's *HIV and AIDS Treatments Directory*.

Are you living well with HIV? and *Feel good, take control, stay healthy*, leaflets produced by the Terrence Higgins Trust.

Nutrition and HIV

A good diet

Having HIV is unlikely to mean that that you have to make any drastic changes to your diet — your existing diet will probably meet all your nutritional needs. A good diet will consist of a balance of the following items:

Starchy food such as bread, cassava, cereals, banana, millet, maizemeal, potatoes, pasta, rice, and yam. Starchy foods should form the basis of your diet, and will provide carbohydrates for energy as well as vitamins, minerals and fibre. You should eat starchy food at every meal, and have four to six portions each day. A portion is equal to one slice of bread, one medium potato, a bowl of cereal or a cup of rice or pasta.

Fruit and vegetables provide vitamins, minerals, fibre and energy. You should eat five portions a day. A portion is equal to a whole piece of fruit, a heaped serving spoon of vegetables, a small glass of fruit juice, or a handful of dried fruit.

Meat, poultry, fish, eggs, beans nuts provide protein, minerals, and vitamins. Try and eat two or three portions per day. A portion is equal to two medium-sized eggs, a 100g piece of meat, a 150g piece of fish, or a small can of baked beans.

Dairy products such as milk, cheese, and yoghurt provide vitamins, minerals and calcium. Three portions should be eaten per day. A portion is equal to a third of a pint of milk, a small pot of yoghurt, or a matchbox-sized piece of cheese.

Fats such cooking oils, butter, margarine, meat and other protein-based foods provide energy, essential fatty acids and the fat-soluble vitamins A, D, E and K. They also provide calcium and phosphate. It is recommended that about a third of your daily calorie intake should come from fats. But be careful. Eating too much fat can lead to weight gain and increased levels of blood fats. This can increase your chance of developing cardiovascular disease and some cancers.

Dietitians

You can obtain advice on your nutritional requirements from a dietitian. Most HIV clinics have specialist dietitians who can:

• Tell you if your existing diet is meeting all your nutritional requirements.

• Give you advice about any changes in your diet that you may need to make.

• Check your body weight and make sure that your proportion of fat to muscle is appropriate.

• Advise you on any dietary changes you may need to make if you are ill.

• Give you advice on food safety.

Dietitians can also assess your body mass index, a guide to whether your height and weight are in proportion.

Supplements

Many people with HIV take dietary supplements, vitamins, or herbal remedies in the hope of boosting or protecting their immune systems and general health.

Evidence that these have any beneficial effect is somewhat thin. What's more, certain supplements, such as large doses of garlic, can stop some anti-HIV drugs working properly. Most HIV specialists would advise that a healthy, balanced diet is enough to meet your nutritional needs. Megadoses of nutritional supplements are not recommended.

Large doses of vitamin A can cause liver and bone damage, as well as vomiting and headache.

Vitamin C doses above 1,000mg per day can cause kidney stones, diarrhoea and the hardening of the arteries, and have been shown to reduce concentrations of the protease inhibitor indinavir (*Crixivan*).

Vitamin E supplements should not be taken if you are taking the protease inhibitor amprenavir (*Agenerase*).

Zinc doses above 75mg per day have been associated with copper deficiencyas well as a shortage of white and/or red blood cells.

Selenium doses of 750 micrograms or more per day have been associated with immune suppression.

Vitamin B6 doses above 2g per day can cause nerve damage, but doses as low as 50mg per day have been known to cause peripheral neuropathy (painful nerve damage), particularly in the feet.

Alcohol in diet

There is no evidence that a couple of alcoholic drinks a day does a person with HIV any harm. Indeed, you might find that a couple of classes of wine or a pint of beer helps reduce stress and anxiety and helps to stimulate your appetite. There's also evidence that a glass or two of alcohol every day can help protect against heart disease.

This isn't an excuse to go out and get roaring drunk every night of the week. Heavy drinking can affect the immune system and slow down recovery from illnesses. Heavy drinking can also cause liver inflammation (hepatitis), and if you have viral hepatitis infections (hepatitis A, hepatitis B, and hepatitis C), you need to talk to your doctor to see if it is safe to drink alcohol at all. The liver plays an important role in processing medicines, particularly drugs used to treat HIV, so it's particularly important to keep your liver healthy if you are HIV-positive.

Alcohol can react badly with some medicines, so whenever you are given a medicine for the first time, ask the pharmacist if it's okay to drink with it.

Food, drink and anti-HIV drugs

Anti-HIV drug combinations may demand one of the following changes to your eating habits:

- Eating at the same time as you take your medication.

- Avoiding food for up to two hours before or an hour after you take your medicines.

- Eating or avoiding certain types of food to ensure that you absorb your medication properly.

When you are prescribed a new medicine, you should be told by your doctor or pharmacist if it has any special dietary restrictions. You should also be given written information explaining what these are.

Detailed information about the dietary restrictions of all the currently available anti-HIV drugs is provided in the NAM booklet *Nutrition*. You can get a free copy from your HIV clinic, or by downloading it from www.aidsmap.com.

Lipodystrophy and diet

Changes in the way the body processes, uses and stores fat have been noticed in some people taking anti-HV drugs. This can lead to changes in body shape or very high levels of blood fats, which can in turn increase the risk of heart disease, stroke and diabetes.

Changes to your diet can help reduce fat levels in your blood (often called lipids). If you are told by your doctor that you have high lipids, try to reduce your intake of saturated fats like dairy products, red meat and animal fats, as well as your sugar and alcohol intake.

Fish oil contains high levels of fatty acids called omega-3 oils, which can reduce fats in the blood. Fish such as mackerel, salmon and trout are a good source. Also, try to make sure that you eat at least five portions of fresh fruit and vegetables a day, as this also protects the heart.

There's a lot more information on lipodystrophy in the chapter *Side-effects*.

Weight loss

When you get ill, you usually lose your appetite. However, when you are ill your nutritional requirements are often increased. Weight loss can be dangerous because it reduces your body's ability to fight off infections and recover.

Dietitians can provide you with some good advice about maintaining your nutritional requirements if you are ill.

Diarrhoea and diet

Diarrhoea is common amongst people with HIV. It can be caused by HIV itself, or by infections or medicines.

Diarrhoea has been reported as a side-effect of all the protease inhibitors, as well as some of the NRTIs and some antibiotics. With some drugs, diarrhoea goes away after the first few weeks of treatment – but some people find that it becomes a permanent feature of living with the drug. The severity of diarrhoea can also differ between people.

Changes of diet seem to have only a limited impact on diarrhoea caused by medicines. But your doctor can prescribe some treatments to help control the diarrhoea. These include:

* Imodium, an anti-diarrhoea drug. It can also be bought over the counter from chemists.

* Calcium supplements have been shown to reduce diarrhoea caused by nelfinavir (*Viracept*).

- Oat bran tablets are also effective against diarrhoea caused by medicines. They work by absorbing fluid and slowing the movement of stool through the gut.

If you have bad diarrhoea, you are likely to lose valuable nutrients. Eating bananas, chicken and fish can help restore levels of potassium which are commonly depleted in people with bad diarrhoea. Avoid coffee, raw vegetables and spicy food as these can make diarrhoea worse.

Further reading

Anti-HIV drugs, and *Nutrition*, booklets in the information for HIV-positive people series produced by NAM.

'A healthy lifestyle' and 'Anti-HIV therapy' in NAM's *HIV and AIDS Treatments Directory*.

Are you living well with HIV? and *Feel good, take control, stay healthy*, leaflets produced by the Terrence Higgins Trust.

Exercise

Benefits of exercise

Everyone can benefit from some form of exercise and experience a lift to their overall health and well-being. Moderate exercise is beneficial to the immune system, and can also improve mood and offer an important way of maintaining a healthy self-image.

Aside from popular forms of exercise like swimming, cycling, aerobics, running and weight training (sometimes called resistance training), there are a number of movement-based exercises, such as yoga, which help maintain muscle tone and suppleness whilst also having meditative or relaxing qualities.

Blood lipids are the name given to fatty substances in the blood, such as cholesterol and triglycerides. Having high levels of these substances in the blood raises your risk of coronary heart disease. Taking anti-HIV drugs may lead to raised blood lipids.

Raising the heart rate for at least thirty minutes three times per week through aerobic exercise (such as cycling, running, swimming, or even brisk walking) reduces these fats, and so lowers risk of heart disease.

People with HIV-related wasting often have low levels of a type of cholesterol called HDL; sometimes referred to as 'good' cholesterol. Resistance training has been shown to significantly increase HDL cholesterol in HIV-positive men with normal testosterone levels.

Regular exercise has been shown to reduce total body and trunk fat among HIV-positive men with body fat changes (lipodystrophy). Resistance exercise reduces raised triglycerides and cholesterol levels.

Planning for exercise

Think about what your aims of exercising are and set yourself some realistic and achievable goals. You may want to get fitter, or you may want to put on weight, lose weight, or achieve a better body shape. Make sure that your aims are achievable – if you're too ambitious you might become disappointed and lose enthusiasm for your exercise programme, or, at worst, injure yourself.

Getting an instructor at a gym to work with you to develop a personal training programme can be a good way of setting yourself achievable goals. Many gyms offer this service as part of an induction package for members. Make sure that you tell the person working with you about any health conditions you have that might make exercise risky (for instance, high blood pressure) or which affect your ability to undertake certain exercises, such as a sprained ankle. There's no reason why you have to tell anybody at a gym or other fitness facility that you are HIV-positive.

Types of exercise

There are two types of exercise. Aerobic exercise (oxygen burning), and resistance (weight training). You're likely to experience the best results with a training programme that incorporates both these types of exercise.

Aerobic exercise

Aerobic exercise improves your heart's ability to pump and your muscles' ability to use oxygen. It includes activities like brisk walking, running, cycling, and swimming.

Aerobic exercise should be strenuous enough to make you out of breath but still able to talk. A total of 30 minutes of aerobic activity per day will reduce your risk of heart disease. If you maintain your heart rate within a training range for 20 to 30 minutes three times a week, you will improve your fitness level. It is easy to calculate your training heart rate. Start by subtracting your age from 220. Then calculate 65% of the resulting figure. This is your optimum training heart rate.

For evample, if you are 54 your training heart rate should be:

• Training HR = 65% of 166 = 108 beats per minute.

Resistance training

The most efficient way to improve your muscle strength and size is through resistance or weight training. Activities like swimming and yoga provide some resistance, but the most efficient way is to use free weights or weight machines at a gym. To improve muscle strength, you need to over-load the muscle. This involves doing quite a small number of repetitions using relatively heavy weights. You should be able to go three sets of 8-12 repetitions. As your strength improves, increase the weight. Always stretch and warm up before exercise. This helps reduce the risk of injury. Don't over-do things. You risk hurting yourself.

People with bleeding disorders should consult their doctor before embarking on a programme of resistance training. Tearing muscles during resistance training can cause internal bleeding that can leave the muscle permanently damaged. People with haemophilia should take Factor VIII if they are weight training.

Sustaining exercise

It's likely that you'll have a high level of enthusiasm when you start your new exercise programme, but this may well diminish in the weeks and months that follow. Exercising can be boring, tiring and uncomfortable. But there are some easy steps you can take to make it easier on yourself:

• It doesn't have to be a chore. Nobody is forcing you to do this. Remember, you are doing it because you want to.

- Choose an exercise activity that you enjoy. There's no point doing something that you don't like. Similarly, if you are going to a gym, choose one that you feel comfortable using.

- Set goals that are achievable, and record your progress.

- Try to prioritise exercise. Don't treat it as a peripheral activity.

- Try and exercise with other people. Becoming a member of a running, swimming or other sporting club can be a great way of exercising with people. Don't feel intimidated – there will be members of all abilities.

- Don't punish yourself or feel guilty if you miss a session or do less than you hoped. You can always go back another day.

- Don't exercise if you are ill or feel unwell. It will probably do you more harm than good.

- Vary your exercise routine.

- Allow yourself regular days off. Your body needs time to recover and benefit from exercise. If you've been exercising regularly, an annual two-week holiday with no exercise won't do you any harm at all.

Fuel for exercise

Before the workout begins, ensure that you are properly hydrated. During each workout, ensure that you maintain an adequate fluid intake. You should try to drink at least 150ml to 250ml every 15 minutes during a session – but if you are taking the protease inhibitor indinavir (*Crixivan*), increase this slightly, to protect against kidney stones.

You're likely to find it uncomfortable if you exercise before breakfast, or immediately after a large meal. The best time to exercise is 30 minutes after a light snack or a meal replacement drink. Do not eat during a workout, but do try to eat a meal high in carbohydrate and protein as soon as possible after each session, in order to promote muscle tissue growth. Seek advice from a registered dietitian at your treatment centre on developing a suitable diet plan.

Steroids

Anabolic steroids can, in certain circumstances (such as severe muscle wasting), be prescribed by your doctor as a way of improving energy levels and enhancing the effects of exercise.

If you have weight loss, anabolic steroids might a way of combating this. Talk to your doctor about whether they would be an appropriate treatment for you.

Many people use anabolic steroids which they have bought illegally, to boost the effects of training at the gym. You should be aware that there are many different kinds of steroids, of differing quality and strength, available, and that inappropriate use can lead to severe liver damage.

Further reading

NAM factsheets, *Cholesterol, Exercise* and *Lipodystrophy*.

Nutrition, booklet in the information for HIV-positive people series produced by NAM.

'A healthy lifestyle' in NAM's *HIV and AIDS Treatments Directory*.

Are you living well with HIV? and *Feel good, take control, stay healthy*, leaflets produced by the Terrence Higgins Trust.

In gear: a gay man's guide to steroids, booklet produced by Camden and Islington's Gay Men's Team, 020 7530 3922.

Travel

Introduction

Being HIV-positive can mean that you need to make detailed plans before travelling. This section provides some general information on how to find out whether a country puts restrictions on entry for people with HIV, and if so, how to deal with these, as well as on travel insurance, vaccinations and receiving medical treatment away from home.

Entry restrictions

Find out if a country you are planning to visit has any entry restrictions for people with HIV. It's generally well known that you cannot visit the USA if you are HIV-positive except in very special circumstances. But other countries also place restrictions on either temporary or long-term visits by individuals with HIV.

The most reliable way of finding out if a country you want to visit restricts entry by people with HIV is to call the embassy or consulate. If you do this, you should not reveal your name or the fact that you are HIV-positive to them. An HIV advocacy or support agency might be willing to do this for you. You might also consider contacting an HIV service organisation in the country you are thinking of traveling to and enquire about entry restrictions. NAM's *AIDS Organisations Worldwide* and *European AIDS Directory* provide listings of major HIV organisations with contact details.

If a country you want to travel to does have entry restrictions, then you need to decide if you want to take the risk of travelling. If you look ill, or are a gay man or an African, you might be more likely to be stopped by customs or immigration, and if they establish that you are HIV-positive, they will probably refuse entry and deport you. Similarly, if you have haemophilia and are travelling with clotting factors or injecting equipment, it's likely that customs officers will question you about your HIV status.

If you are a citizen of an EU country, or have the right to live in an EU country, then there should be no restrictions on your admittance to another EU member state. But because you receive free HIV care in the UK doesn't necessarily mean that you will be entitled to it in the country you are visiting.

If you are planning a long-term visit or permanent move to another country, make sure at a very early stage in your planning that your HIV status isn't going to be a problem. A good place to start would be to contact an HIV service organisation in the country you want to move to. NAM's *AIDS Organisations Worldwide* and *European AIDS Directory* list major organisations that you might want to consider contacting.

Travelling with medication

If you are taking anti-HIV drugs you'll need to carry them with them when you travel. Customs officials often take a particular interest in medicines, and the discovery of anti-HIV drugs in the luggage of people with HIV has been the reason why many people have been refused entry to the USA and deported.

Some people get around the risk of travelling with their medication by taking the following action:

- They send their medication in advance. But make sure it arrives before you travel. Remember, post can be inspected by customs.

- Obtain medication in the country you want to travel to. However, this may not always be possible – or it could be extremely expensive.

If you carry your medication with you, have an answer ready about what the drugs are for. Some people say they are for cancer treatment. But remember, there's a reasonable chance that a customs official will have seen anti-HIV drugs before and won't be easily fooled. It might be helpful to have a letter from your doctor saying that the medicines you are carrying are for the treatment of a chronic medical condition and are for personal use. Make sure the letter doesn't mention HIV.

It might be very difficult, or even impossible, to get supplies of your medication once you've left home – even if you are just taking a short trip in the UK or Europe. So make sure you take enough of all your medicines with you to last the full duration of your trip. It might be wise to count out your medicines before you travel and to take a few additional doses just in case you get delayed.

Travelling across international time zones is likely to have implications for the time you take your medication. There are three options you may wish to consider. These include continuing to take your medicines at your UK time – but this could mean that you have to take your doses at inconvenient times. Another option is to gradually adjust the time you take your medicines, from UK time to the time in the country you are visiting. A third option might be altering your dose time to fit in with the time zone of the country you are visiting, but this could mean that there are some long intervals between doses as you adjust. It might be wise to talk over your plan with a doctor or pharmacist before you travel.

In good enough health to travel?

If you are planning a trip, then the chances are that your health will be up to it. But if you are feeling unwell, ask yourself honestly if you are in sufficiently good health to travel. Being ill away from home can be, at the very least, inconvenient, and it might be difficult to obtain specialist medical care or to come home early. What's more, if you are very ill, some airlines might refuse to carry you.

Travel insurance

General travel insurance policies generally exclude cover for pre-existing medical conditions, and some specifically exclude HIV. However it might be worth taking out cover just in case you have an illness that is unrelated to HIV, have an accident, lose your luggage or have something stolen.

What's more, some insurance companies are now willing to provide cover for people with HIV. Restrictions tend to apply, and premiums are often inflated.

NAM cannot recommend any particular provider of travel insurance company. It might be wise to shop around for a range of quotes and select the insurer which most meets your specific needs.

Freedom Travel Insurance

0870 774 3760

www.tht.org.uk/freedom_insurance/freedom01.htm

Easy Travel Insurance

0870 345 345

www.hivtravelinsurance.com

Rothwell and Towler

01404 41234

www.travelfirst.co.uk

Reciprocal medical care

If you are travelling to another EU country you should obtain an E111 certificate before you travel. This will provide you with free or reduced cost medical care in EU and some other countries. You can obtain this from a Post Office. The form will tell you the exact treatment which individual countries offer under the scheme. You may not get free medical treatment in some countries.

Vaccinations

Find out if you need any special vaccinations and if it is safe for you to receive them. Generally, people with HIV should not be given 'live' vaccines. Talk to your doctor.

Treatment breaks and travel

Do not take a break from your HIV treatments or any other medicines you have been prescribed without discussing it with your doctor in advance.

Further reading

NAM factsheets, *Travelling with your HIV drugs* and *Treatment interruption*.

'Travel' in NAM's *AIDS Reference Manual* (last updated in June 2003).

An up-to-date list of countries which impose restrictions on HIV-positive travellers can be found at this website: http://www.aidsnet.ch/.

Holiday hassles and HRT, by Caroline Guinness

A much-needed holiday. Tickets, passports, driving licence – all go in my hand luggage. I leave the toiletry bag out till the last minute. I don't care if everything else gets lost, but those pills must come with me on the plane. Into the bag they go.

The taxi's here right on time. Easy check-in at Gatwick, time to buy a few duty frees, which I've left space for in my hand luggage...I open it...stab of ice-cold fear...the toiletry bag...at home!

"Oh my God!" Husband goes pale. "Do you want to go back ?" A few seconds' hesitation – "No! I'm getting on that plane."

A frantic call on the mobile (didn't forget that!) to the travel agent. No more flights till next week. FedEx will not courier medicines. A friend at home will try other courier companies.

I call my clinic. No, they do not know any doctors in Lanzarote but they will fax a letter and prescription to the travel rep there. I call the travel agent for their fax number. It turns out they are also the car hire company at Lanzarote Airport. My friend calls back, she has found a courier but the pills will have to go via Madrid and will not reach me till Monday (it is now Thursday). Our flight is being called.

Sitting on the plane, I realise that the travel rep and the car hire person will now know that I am HIV-positive. Oh great. In addition, I do not have my HRT – hormone hell for me and hubby, not a good prospect!

We land, find rep, she is fantastic. Married to a local doctor, she has spent the last two hours trying to sort things out – no go. The clinic system is like the UK – they

don't just hand over HIV pills willy-nilly. She takes me to
the airport pharmacy. A sweet man hands over my HRT,
which is a major relief, but no HIV combo.

Weather perfect, accommodation divine. I call my clinic,
they tell me not to panic, things should be OK. I have been
adherent for four years, undetectable and feeling well. There
might be a small 'blip'. Just make sure to take my pills as
soon as they arrive, make sure I have bloods done as soon
as I return. I have done everything I can.

I do not feel stressed. In fact, I feel fantastic. Have my first
good night's sleep in years. Have my first 'real' dreams.
Wake up refreshed for the first time in years. Husband says
he can see my shoulders dropping. I feel light and
NORMAL.

Monday, I call Madrid. My pills have left there and are on
their way to Las Palmas, then another flight to Lanzarote,
and should be there by 4.15pm. I do not feel relieved.
Strangely sad, in fact.

"Why?" my husband asks.

"Well, let me try and explain. Imagine you lost a leg and
were given an artificial one. You are grateful for the
mobility it gives you. Then for four days your leg grows
back, but only for four days. Does that make it clearer?"

Pills in my hand, swallow. Within two hours I am feeling
weird, slight hallucinations, sick. That night 'the dreams'.
Wake feeling vile. How come? The sun is still shining, I'm
still on holiday. Yet that low level of anxiety is back. Now I
know it's not me, it's the efavirenz.

I know what it is to have AIDS; I know these things are a
better alternative. I should be grateful, but still I grieve. I
realise, now, why we are entitled to Disability Living
Allowance. You may not see the disability, but this is what
it feels like. It's real.

A week later, I am back at my Clinic. "How do you feel?" They ask anxiously. "Fine," I reply. "You look great." I always do with a suntan!

I see my consultant on 20th March. No viral 'blip', thank God, but psychologically, it has not just been a 'blip', it's been an explosion. I must discuss (again) a Structured Treatment Interruption. Oh for a cure!

This first appeared in issue 78 of Positive Nation, May 2002. Many thanks to both Caroline and Positive Nation for giving permission to reprint it.

Sex and HIV

Introduction

The overwhelming majority of people with HIV remain sexually active after they find out they have HIV. For most people, sex is a pleasurable and important part of life, and many people with HIV have sex that they are happy with.

Nevertheless, it's important for people with HIV to have information about sex and their health. This chapter provides information on what's involved in protecting your own and other people's sexual health, sexual problems such as erectile dysfunction, infectiousness, and reinfection with other strains of HIV.

Protecting your own and other people's health

It's a pretty obvious point, but one worth making nevertheless: HIV can be passed on to another person during sex.

Each individual needs to make their own decisions about the steps they are willing to take (and practically can take) to prevent them passing on HIV to another person.

Ultimately, it's a personal decision, which is likely to be influenced by a whole host of individual circumstances.

Nevertheless, it's important to be aware that if you have unprotected sex with a person who is HIV-negative (whether you know this or not), and they are infected with HIV by you, there could be serious legal consequences. In both England and Scotland HIV-positive men have been jailed after failing to tell their female sex partners they were HIV-positive and infecting them with HIV. This issue is looked at in more detail in the section on the law and HIV. In some other countries, most notably some states of the USA, it is a crime for an HIV-positive individual to have sex with another person without disclosing their HIV status.

There are other factors which you might also wish to have in mind when making decisions about sex. Unprotected sex carries the risk of acquiring sexually transmitted infections, which can be unpleasant. The viruses hepatitis B and hepatitis C can be sexually transmitted and can have very serious health consequences. Pregnancy is another obvious risk for women of child-bearing age. There's also some evidence that people with HIV can in some circumstances be reinfected with another strain of HIV which might be more difficult to treat.

These issues are considered in more detail below.

Disclosing your HIV status to partners

The bottom line is that there's no legal requirement in the UK to tell your sexual partners that you're HIV-positive. It's up to you. Some individuals always disclose their HIV status, others never do. It's very much a personal choice, influenced by individual circumstances.

If you do feel that you want to tell your past, current, or future sexual partners that you have HIV, then think about how you are going to do this, and think how you might respond to their reactions, which might not be what you hoped for. Health advisers at sexual health clinics can contact your ex-partners for you (if you are willing for them to do this and it is practical).

Anal and vaginal sex

Unprotected anal and vaginal sex are the types of sex which carry the greatest risk of HIV transmission. Oral sex is considered in detail in a section below.

The chances of you passing on HIV during unprotected anal or vaginal sex are greatest if you are the active, or insertive, partner during sex. The risk is particularly high if you have a high viral load or an untreated STI, or if you ejaculate inside your partner. Similarly, if an HIV-negative person has an untreated STI, their chances of contracting HIV from you during unprotected sex are increased.

If you are HIV-positive and are the passive, or receptive, partner during insertive sex, the risk of you passing on HIV is reduced, but is still present, especially if you have an untreated STI.

Unprotected vaginal sex also carries the risk of pregnancy. Emergency contraception is available from clinics and from pharmacies without prescription.

Oral sex

The risk of transmitting HIV by oral sex is much less certain. The UK body which monitors rates of HIV estimates that about 1-3% of all sexual transmission of HIV is due to oral sex.

However, the evidence is conflicting, with some doctors and studies suggesting that as many as 8% of HIV infections are due to oral sex, and others putting the figure much lower, even at zero.

It seems that if there is a risk from oral sex, it is much lower than the risk from unprotected anal or vaginal sex. Having a very high viral load, an untreated STI, ejaculating in the mouth of the person sucking and the presence of sores or wounds in the mouth of the person sucking seem to increase the risk.

Condoms

Condoms can prevent you from getting most STIs and can stop you passing on HIV to other people or being reinfected with another strain of HIV. Condoms only work when used properly.

In the UK and some other countries, extra-strong condoms used to be recommended for anal sex, but recent research has found that standard strength condoms are just as safe. A water-based lubricant should be used with condoms, as oil-based ones weaken the rubber in condoms and can cause tiny tears. Condoms should never be reused.

If you are having sex for a long time, then it is safest to change condoms.

HIV and sexual health clinics provide free condoms, and in some cities free condoms can also be obtained from gay venues. They can also be obtained from family planning clinics.

Condoms should be disposed of as rubbish and not flushed down the toilet.

Use of anti-HIV drugs to prevent infection with HIV

If a person thinks that they have been exposed to HIV during sex, many clinics are willing to provide them with a short-course of anti-HIV drugs to try to prevent infection. This is called post-exposure prophylaxis, or PEP for short. However, not all clinics offer it for sexual exposure, because of worries about side-effects and resistance. Nevertheless, it is becoming more widely available. PEP is not a kind of "morning-after pill" for HIV and it's not 100% effective.

PEP may also be considered in cases of rape and sexual assault where there is a risk of HIV transmission.

It is important to provide PEP as soon as possible after possible exposure to HIV — ideally within four hours, and certainly within 72 hours.

Sexual health check-ups

If you are sexually active, it is wise to have regular sexual health check-ups, every three months or so. These are free and confidential. Many HIV clinics have sexual health clinics (sometimes called GUM clinics) attached, and some HIV clinics now include sexual health screens as part of their routine HIV care. However, you can choose which sexual health clinic you go to.

Most people with HIV in the UK were diagnosed through sexual health clinics, so you may already know what services they provide.

Visits to sexual health clinics normally involve seeing a doctor or nurse who will ask you about the kind of sex you are having and examine you for symptoms. It is important to be honest if you have had unprotected sex so you can have the appropriate tests. Sexual health clinics should be very used to seeing all the communities affected by HIV in the UK, including gay men and Africans, and their services should be non-judgmental.

Check-ups normally involve having swabs taken from the tip of the penis or inside the vagina and from the mouth and throat and anus if you have had oral or anal sex. You will also be asked to provide a urine sample. These samples are then examined under a microscope or cultured to see if any bacteria grows.

Blood samples are also taken, to check for other infections. Some results can be given to you at the time of your visit, but it may be necessary to telephone or call back a week or so later for some other results.

All treatment for STIs at NHS sexual health clinics is free of charge.

If you have an STI, you may be offered the opportunity to see a health adviser. Health advisers can give you information about STIs and how to avoid them and can help you contact your sexual partners, if this is possible or practical and you agree, so they can be tested and treated. Health advisers can also offer referrals to other specialist services.

Sexually transmitted infections

Bacteria and viruses can cause sexually transmitted infections (STIs). Mites that burrow under the skin, called scabies, can also be passed on during sex, as can pubic lice (crabs). Bacterial infections can be cured with antibiotics, and antiviral drugs can be used to treat some of the viral infections. Lotions can clear infestations of scabies and lice.

This section gives a brief explanation of the ways in which common STIs and infestations are passed on, their symptoms, and their treatment.

Chlamydia
Transmission

Chlamydia can be transmitted during anal, oral and vaginal sex if no condom is used, and can affect the anus, penis, cervix, throat and eyes.

Symptoms

Symptoms of chlamydia normally occur one to three weeks after infection. However, many people who have chlamydia are unaware that they have the infection. It is thought that as many as 75 per cent of women and 50 per cent of men with chlamydia have no symptoms.

Where symptoms do occur, in men they usually consist of a milky discharge from the penis, particularly in the morning, and a burning sensation when urinating. Chlamydia can also cause the testicles to swell. If a person has been infected anally, there may be soreness around the anus and a discharge.

Women with chlamydia may notice a milky discharge from the vagina and/or lower abdominal or back pain, or pain when having sex. There may also be vaginal bleeding during sex and bleeding between periods.

If chlamydia is left untreated it can lead to pelvic inflammatory disease (PID) in women, which can cause ectopic pregnancy, infertility, and even death in extreme cases. Men are less likely to develop serious complications, though untreated chlamydia may cause infertility. Both men and women may develop arthritis as a consequence of untreated chlamydia.

Diagnosis

Chlamydia is diagnosed by taking a swab from the penis or cervix. This can be a little uncomfortable, but is usually very quick. Some clinics also examine a urine sample for evidence of infection with chlamydia.

It can, however, take up to a week for tests to show if chlamydia is present and it is important to contact your clinic for the result of your test so treatment can be given if the infection has been detected.

Treatment

Chlamydia is treated with antibiotics. Normally this consists of a seven-day course of doxycycline, or a single dose of azithromycin. It is important to take all your tablets to ensure that the infection is eradicated from your body. It's also important to try and ensure that your partner receives treatment. Symptoms may persist for a few days after taking azithromycin, as the antibiotic takes time to work.

You may be asked to return a week later for a test to see if your treatment has been effective. You are likely to be advised not to have sex (even with a condom) until your treatment period is finished. This is to prevent re-infection.

Genital warts
Transmission

Genital warts are a sexually transmitted infection caused by the human papilloma virus and are the commonest STI in the UK. They can be contracted during unprotected anal, vaginal or oral sex. They can also be transmitted by close physical contact with the genital warts themselves, as these may shed the wart virus.

Symptoms

Genital warts look just like warts which may appear on other parts of the body – usually small lumps on the skin with a slightly rough texture. Some people who contract the wart virus do not have symptoms, however, or else do not notice the presence of warts. In women, warts may appear on the inside or outside of the vagina, or on the neck of the cervix or around the anus. In men, warts may appear on the tip or shaft of the penis or around the anus.

Some forms of the genital warts virus are associated with an increased risk of cervical or anal cancer, and this risk might be increased even further in people with HIV. However, these are not the most common form of the wart virus.

Diagnosis

Genital warts are diagnosed by visual and manual examination of the genital and anal area.

A PAP smear is a procedure designed to detect pre-cancerous cellular changes called dysplasia early, before cancer develops. Most women know the PAP smear as a cervical smear. PAP smears involve taking a small scraping of cells from the cervix. When these cells are examined under a microscope, it is possible to see if there are any changes in the cells which suggest a risk that cancer could develop in the future.

HIV-positive women are recommended to have PAP smears when they are first diagnosed with HIV, six months later, and then at least once a year. The value of screening the anal canal for pre-cancerous cells is being studied.

Treatment

Infection with the genital wart virus is cured by your own immune system and this can take a long time. Treatment to remove the visible warts involves either painting the warts with a chemical that burns them, freezing, laser surgery or a new immune stimulating cream. Some of these procedures may be a little uncomfortable.

Gonorrhoea

Gonorrhoea is a bacterial STI that can be passed on during anal, vaginal, oral and mouth-to-anus (rimming) sex. Gonorrhoea can affect the anus, penis, cervix and throat. Untreated gonorrhoea can make a person with HIV more infectious. Having gonorrhoea can also make it more likely that an HIV-negative person will be infected if they are exposed to the virus. Gonorrhoea can also be passed on from mother to baby during childbirth, and can cause infection in the baby's eyes, resulting in blindness if left untreated.

Symptoms

Symptoms of gonorrhoea usually appear between two and ten days after infection. However, some people may not realise they have the infection as symptoms may not always be present, or may be mild. In men, symptoms usually consist of a yellowish or greenish discharge from the penis and burning when passing urine. The testicles may also hurt and swell.

Symptoms in women can include a burning sensation when passing urine and a discoloured or bloody discharge from the vagina. If the infection is rectal, both men and women may notice a mucousy or bloody discharge from the anus, pain in the anus, or pain when having anal sex. Gonorrhoea in the throat can cause a sore throat, but usually doesn't.

If left untreated, gonorrhoea can cause more serious health problems, including pelvic infections in women, resulting in pain, infertility, and ectopic pregnancy, and testicular problems in men.

Untreated gonorrhoea can also spread to the bloodstream, leading to fevers, and can affect the joints, causing arthritic-like pain and swelling.

Diagnosis

To test for gonorrhoea, a swab is taken from the tip of the penis or from the cervix. If you have told the doctor that you have had oral or anal sex, swabs will also be taken from the throat and/or anus. The swabs can be a little uncomfortable. A urine sample may also be taken. It is usually possible to tell immediately from examination of the swabs if gonorrhoea is present in the penis, and in many cases the cervix, but gonorrhoea in the throat can usually only be diagnosed later. However, whatever the site of infection, it can take up to three days for testing to provide conclusive results. It is important, therefore, to contact your clinic for the result of your test so treatment can be given if the bacteria have been detected.

Treatment

Gonorrhoea is treated with antibiotics. These are normally given by injection.

You will be asked to return seven days later for tests to see that you have been cured. You are likely to be advised not to have sex (even with a condom) until your treatment period is finished. This is to prevent reinfection.

Hepatitis A
Transmission

Hepatitis A is a virus which affects the liver and is transmitted through contact with infected faeces (excrement, shit), normally in contaminated food. However, it can be passed on during sex, particularly oral-anal (rimming) contact. There have been outbreaks of hepatitis A amongst gay men in several cities in recent years. Once you have had hepatitis A, you cannot get it again.

Symptoms

Hepatitis A can cause a short-term mild illness, and symptoms can include a yellowing of the skin and eyes (jaundice), extreme tiredness, weight loss, vomiting, diarrhoea, dark urine and pale stools. Symptoms can be made worse by drinking alcohol, tea or coffee or by eating fatty food. People normally get better after a couple of weeks.

Diagnosis

Sexual health clinics do not routinely test for hepatitis A, but blood tests can be used to detect the virus, as can examination of stool samples.

Treatment

Treatment for hepatitis A consists of rest, drinking fluids, and avoiding alcohol and recreational drugs. It's also important not to take paracetamol while you are recovering from hepatitis A. Hepatitis A can last longer and be more severe in people with HIV and weakened immune systems. If you have hepatitis A it might be necessary to stop taking anti-HIV drugs for a time, as most medicines are broken down by the liver – and when the liver is inflamed by hepatitis A, side-effects can become worse.

Vaccination

A vaccination is available for hepatitis A, and everybody with HIV is recommended to have it if they do not have natural immunity to the infection. The vaccination consists of two injections given over a number of months.

Hepatitis B
See the section on hepatitis B in the chapter *Symptoms and illnesses*.

Hepatitis C
See the section on hepatitis C in the chapter *Symptoms and illnesses*.

Herpes
An outbreak of herpes involves painful sores or ulcers that affect the mouth or genitals. Herpes is caused by a common virus called herpes simplex virus (HSV).

Once you are infected, the virus stays in skin and nerve cells for life. However, you may not know that you are infected with HSV. Most of the time it is dormant and causes no symptoms. From time to time, flare-ups occur, especially if you have a weakened immune system. Even among people without HIV, stress, a common cold or exposure to strong ultra-violet light can cause an outbreak of active herpes.

There are two main types of HSV. HSV-1 usually causes oral herpes, or cold sores – tingling or painful spots on the edge of the lip where it meets the skin of the face. These can occasionally develop on the nostrils, on the gums or on the roof of the mouth.

HSV-2 is the usual cause of genital herpes – painful genital or anal ulcers, sometimes accompanied by fever, headache, muscle ache and malaise. Herpes lesions often start as numbness, tingling or itching. This feeling indicates that the virus is travelling up a nerve to the skin. There it causes small bumps that rapidly develop into small, inflamed, fluid-filled blisters. These burst and crust over, typically taking one or two weeks to heal in people with normal immune systems.

Transmission

The virus can be passed from person to person by contact between these lesions and mucous membranes e.g. by kissing, and sexual contact.

Herpes may also be transmitted when sores are not present, if HSV is replicating and infectious HSV particles are being shed from the skin or, more likely, from mucous membranes. HIV-positive people may experience such shedding more frequently.

There is evidence that recent infection with genital herpes ulcers substantially increases the chances of a person being infected with HIV.

In people with HIV, herpes recurrences tend to be more frequent, more severe and longer lasting. Sometimes the lesions can become infected with other bacteria or fungi. As well as causing large oral and genital lesions, herpes can occasionally affect the throat, colon and other organs, including the liver, eye and lung.

Diagnosis

HSV is diagnosed by growing (culturing) the virus from a swab taken from a lesion, or by using a fluorescent screening test to detect the virus. A test that looks directly for the genetic material of the virus is used for research purposes but is not generally available. Herpes in the oesophagus (gullet) or colon may be examined using fibre-optic instruments.

Treatment and preventing recurrance

Herpes infections are treated with aciclovir. Other treatments for herpes include valaciclovir, and famciclovir.

Aciclovir is taken in tablet form (200-800 mg fives times a day for 5 – 10 days) to treat serious attacks of oral herpes and genital or anal ulcers. Although it is effective at preventing outbreaks of herpes, once an attack of genital herpes is established, aciclovir often provides minimal benefit. It is also given as an intravenous drip (5 – 10 mg/kg every 8 hours) for very severe attacks. Aciclovir has very few side-effects. Aciclovir cannot eliminate HSV virus in nerve cells, so herpes attacks may recur after an attack has been treated. Aciclovir cream is available from chemists to treat cold sores; however, many doctors question its efficacy.

Aciclovir may be taken on a regular basis to prevent recurrent attacks of herpes (400mg twice daily). Some people also find that salt baths relieve symptoms.

Non-specific urethritis (NSU)
Transmission

Non-specific urethritis (NSU) affects only men and is an inflammation of theurethra – the tube which urine and semen pass through in a man's penis. This inflammation can be caused by several infections transmitted during unprotected anal, oral, or vaginal sex. However, very rarely it can have a non-sexual cause, such as friction during sex.

Symptoms

Symptoms of NSU normally develop within a week or so of infection, although some irritants, such as soap, can cause symptoms to occur almost immediately. However, it is estimated that as many as 50% of men with NSU have no symptoms at all.

When symptoms do occur, they normally consist of pain or a burning sensation when passing urine, a white or cloudy discharge from the tip of the penis, which may be particularly noticeable first thing in the morning, and more frequent urination.

Diagnosis

NSU is diagnosed by taking a swab from the penis. This can be uncomfortable but is very quick to take. A urine sample may also be looked at for evidence of infection.

In many cases it will be possible to tell instantly if NSU is present, but it can take up to a week for tests to show if chlamydia, the symptoms of which can resemble NSU, is present.

Treatment

NSU is treated with antibiotics. Normally this consists of a seven-day course of doxycycline or a single dose of azithromycin. It is important to take all your tablets to ensure that the infection has been eradicated from your body. Symptoms may persist for a few days after taking azithromycin, as the antibiotic takes time to work.

You may be asked to return a week later for a test to see that you have been cured. You are likely to be advised not to have sex (even with a condom) until your treatment period has finished. Your partner should, whereever possible, also receive treatment. This is to prevent re-infection.

Pubic lice (crabs)
Transmission

Pubic lice are small insects that resemble crabs because of their claws, which allow them to hold onto pubic hair (body hair near the genitals and anus). Although crabs are particularly fond of pubic hair, they can live in hair in other parts of the body, particularly the armpits, and even in the eyebrows and eyelashes, although this is uncommon.

Crabs are normally picked up and passed on during sex, though any form of intimate bodily contact can be enough to pass them on. They can also be picked up from sharing towels, bedding or clothing, but this is less common.

Symptoms and diagnosis

Some people notice the infestation within hours, but others do not become aware that they have crabs for several weeks. Crabs are very small and can be very difficult to see, but symptoms usually include an intense itching in the groin, and some people notice the lice eggs firmly attached to pubic hair. Small spots of blood may appear on underwear or sheets.

Treatments

Lotions such as *Derbac* are available from chemists, without prescription, for getting rid of crabs, and these are also available free of charge from sexual health and GUM clinics. It is important to follow the instructions properly as improper use could mean that you fail to clear the infestation, and using too much could provoke an allergic reaction. Do not use Derbac or similar lotions after a hot bath.

Shaving pubic hair will not get rid of crabs. It is important to wash all clothes, towels and bedding you have used since you picked up crabs on a hot cycle when you start treatment. You should also ensure that your partner, or people with whom you have shared a bed or had intimate bodily contact, has treatment at the same time as you to avoid reinfestation.

Scabies
Transmission

Scabies is a skin disease caused by a mite that burrows under the skin, causing intense itching that is usually most notable at night.

It is easy to pick up scabies – any skin contact is enough, and sharing towels or bedding is enough for transmission to occur.

Symptoms

Scabies are invisible to the naked eye, but leave red 'track marks' in the skin. Usually scabies affect the hands between the fingers, the genitals, breasts, buttocks, abdomen and feet.

Treatment

The same lotions used to treat crab infestations are also effective against scabies, although it may be necessary to leave the lotion on the body for longer (usually 24 hours). It should be applied to the whole body, other than the face and scalp, and reapplied to the hands after hand-washing if this is an area of infestation. After treatment, the itch can get worse temporarily. In this case, hydrocortisone cream can be applied, and the itch should not be scratched.

Clothing, towels and bedding should be washed on a hot cycle to avoid infecting others or yourself. As with crabs, it is important that anybody who you think might have been infested at the same time as you, and with whom you are in intimate contact, treats themselves at the same time as you to avoid reinfestation.

Neither scabies nor crabs can pass on HIV. People with long-standing crab infestations can feel generally unwell (which is the origin of the term lousy) and if left untreated, scabies can cause severe skin irritation.

Syphilis

Syphilis is a complex infection caused by bacteria. The number of cases in the UK and many other countries has increased dramatically in recent years. There are three stages to the disease: primary syphilis, secondary syphilis and tertiary syphilis. During the primary and secondary stages, the disease is highly contagious.

Transmission

Syphilis can be contracted from contact with syphilitic sores during unprotected anal, oral or vaginal sex. It can also be transmitted by close physical contact with syphilitic rashes and lesions, which can be anywhere on the body, and from contact with blood. Syphilis can also be transmitted from mother to baby.

It's likely that untreated primary and secondary syphilis can make a person with HIV more infectious. Having syphilis may also make it much more likely that an HIV-negative person will be infected with HIV if exposed to the virus.

Symptoms

Syphilis can cause a range of symptoms or none at all. In the early stage of disease, symptoms may be easily missed. Syphilis can progress more quickly and severely in people with HIV, and may present slightly different symptoms.

Shortly after becoming infected with syphilis (primary syphilis), a small sore, spot or ulcer (called a chancre) may appear at the site of infection, usually on the penis, in or around the anus or vagina or in the mouth. The chancre does not hurt and usually heals quite quickly. It can be accompanied by swollen glands.

Secondary syphilis can cause a rash, swollen glands, fever, muscle pain, headache, ringing in the ears, and in rare cases, meningitis. Dark brown sores, about the size of a penny piece, may also appear on the hands and feet. The rash and sores are highly infectious. Secondary syphilis normally develops within six months of exposure.

Tertiary syphilis usually develops within ten years of infection and can cause damage to almost all the internal organs and the brain (neurosyphilis). If left untreated, syphilis can cause death.

Diagnosis

A general sexual health check-up will include a blood test for syphilis, and any lesions will be swabbed. Many HIV clinics now test for syphilis as part of their routine HIV care. It can take up to three months for the body to develop antibodies to the bacteria that cause syphilis, so a test taken shortly after exposure may not detect infection. There is some evidence to suggest that tests for syphilis are not as reliable in HIV-positive people. If brain involvement is suspected, a lumbar puncture may be carried out to assess the extent of disease.

Treatment

Syphilis is usually treated with a course of penicillin injections. People who are allergic to penicillin are given a course of antibiotic tablets. To ensure that the syphilis is completely cured, it is vital to have all your prescribed injections or take all your medication. To avoid infecting other people with syphilis, or being re-infected with the bacteria, it is important to avoid sex altogether until treatment has been completed and you have been given the all-clear.

Follow-up blood tests will be carried out at intervals of 1, 2, 3, 6, 12 and 24 months to ensure the infection has gone.

Trichomonas

Trichomonas vaginalis is a common sexually transmitted infection caused by a tiny parasite.

Transmission

Trichomonas is spread by unprotected sex between men and women.

Symptoms

In women, symptoms can include a smelly vaginal discharge, vaginal itching, lower back pain, pain during sex and a frequent need to urinate. Often men have no symptoms, but when they do, a discharge from the penis, a burning pain when urinating and an increased need to urinate are most common.

Diagnosis

Swabs taken from the vagina or penis are examined for the presence of trichomonas under a microscope, and it is often possible to tell immediately if infection is present. Swabs can also be cultured, with results available in a week.

Treatment

Trichomonas is treated with antibiotics. It is important to take all your tablets to ensure that the infection has been eradicated from your body. You may be asked to return a week later for a test to see that you have been cured. You are likely to be advised not to have sex (even with a condom) until your treatment period has finished. This is to prevent re-infection.

Other infections

Other infections can also be spread during sex. Any sex which involves contact with faeces, even in microscopic amounts, such as rimming and anal sex and fisting, can lead to the transmission of gut infections such as giardia and *cryptosporidiosis*. These can cause bad diarrhoea and vomiting, which needs to be treated with antibiotics.

Undetectable viral load and infectiousness

An undetectable HIV viral load is the goal of anti-HIV treatment. This does not mean that a person has been cured of HIV, but rather that the combination of drugs a person is taking has reduced HIV's ability to reproduce so it can no longer be detected in the blood.

An undetectable viral load in blood does not necessarily mean that a person is not infectious. Although many people with undetectable viral loads in their blood also have an undetectable viral load in their semen and seem less likely to transmit HIV, this is not always the case. Some people with undetectable viral loads in their blood have quite high viral loads in their sexual fluids, which could be high enough to infect somebody else.

Studies have mainly been conducted in men, and these have found that having an untreated STI, particularly gonorrhoea, increases the chances that viral load will be detectable in semen.

In addition, studies have found that a small number of men with high blood viral loads have very high viral loads in their semen and are very infectious.

Also, if a person is resistant to anti-HIV drugs, they can infect other people with drug-resistant HIV. About 10% of new HIV-infections in the UK are with drug-resistant virus. This means that the person newly infected with HIV already has limited treatment options before they have taken a single anti-HIV drug.

Reinfection

In addition to STIs, unprotected sex can have other health risks for HIV-positive people. There have been cases reported where a person with HIV has been reinfected, or 'superinfected', with another subtype or strain of HIV which is resistant to anti-HIV drugs.

In some cases, this has resulted in the person's HIV viral load increasing and CD4 cell count falling. In addition, their treatment options have been limited because the type of HIV they were reinfected with was resistant to some or all of the anti-HIV drugs they were taking – and to others they had never taken.

It is not known how easy it is for somebody to become reinfected with HIV. So far, only a few cases have been reported worldwide, almost all amongst gay men who had unprotected anal sex. However, there has also been a case reported of reinfection involving a heterosexual couple.

Although reinfection appears to be rare, there seem to be some factors that might increase the risk of it happening. The main one appears to be taking a break from treatment. The reasons for this are not fully understood.

Pregnancy and conception

Because of successful anti-HIV treatments, and the availability of effective means of reducing the risk of mother-to-baby transmission of HIV, many HIV-positive women have reconsidered their decisions about sex, relationships and having children.

If you would like support to think through these issues, it may be helpful to see a counsellor, or to talk to other HIV-positive women. One option is Positively Women, a national organisation providing peer support to HIV-positive women. Their telephone number is 020 7713 0222. Another organisation is Body and Soul, a self-help organisation which supports women, heterosexual men, children and families living with or affected by HIV. You can telephone them on 020 7383 768.

In the UK, HIV treatment centres provide condoms free of charge. The NHS also provides free access to contraceptives. Contraception is available from GPs and family planning clinics. Details of family planning clinics are available from NHS Direct on 0845 46 47.

If you are thinking of becoming pregnant, it's very important that you tell your doctor so they can, with you, reduce the risks of your baby being infected with HIV. The use of anti-HIV drugs during pregnancy, choosing a caesarian delivery and not breastfeeding can mean that an HIV-positive mother can have an HIV-negative baby. For more information on preventing mother-to-baby transmission of HIV see the chapter *Mother-to-baby transmission of HIV*.

If you are an HIV-negative woman with an HIV-positive male partner and wish to become pregnant, one option you may want to consider is sperm washing. Using this technique, semen can be `washed' by separating sperm and seminal fluid; the sperm sample is then incubated to allow live sperm to separate from dead sperm, and this sample can then be used for insemination.

So far there have been no cases of HIV transmission to the female partner using this method. Unfortunately, few centres in the UK offer this service and NHS funding remains limited. This method has been under investigation at the Chelsea and Westminster Hospital in London since 1999.

A woman wishing to conceive by this method will be monitored to determine when she is due to ovulate, and then her partner will be asked to provide a sperm sample which is washed before testing it for HIV. If the sample is negative, the insemination can proceed. The Chelsea and Westminster Hospital warns couples wanting to undertake the process that even after washing, around 5-6% of samples have tested HIV-positive.

So far, dozens of HIV-1 positive men with HIV-negative partners have been treated at the Chelsea and Westminster Hospital. Following a sexual health and fertility screen on each partner, sperm washing was performed with intrauterine insemination (IUI). If a fertility problem is diagnosed, the couples receive IVF treatment.

Ongoing pregnancy/live birth rates per cycle were 10.6% (10/94) for IUI and 23.8% (10/42) for IVF. Many healthy children have been born, with no cases of HIV infection in either the women or their infants. However, there is little NHS funding available for sperm washing and one cycle of IUI costs several hundred pounds.

Sexual problems

While sexual dysfunction can be a problem for anyone, people living with HIV may be particularly affected. Loss of sexual drive or desire (libido) can have a significant impact on quality of life and feelings of self-worth, and may even contribute to emotional problems such as anxiety and depression

Sexual problems are common during times of stress, such as when one receives an HIV-positive diagnosis or experiences work or relationship difficulties. Excessive intake of alcohol or recreational drugs can also diminish both the desire and ability to have sex.

Many of the drugs commonly used to treat depression, e.g. fluoxetine (*Prozac*) or paroxetine (*Seroxat*) can also affect sexual function. Additionally, megestrol acetate (*Megace*), an appetite stimulant, has been shown to cause loss of libido.

Sexual dysfunction among men can often be a result of decreased testosterone levels (hypogonadism), which can also lead to fatigue. Lower than normal testosterone levels have been found in people with advanced HIV infection, and can be caused both by the direct effects of HIV or simply by chronic ill health. Many men receive testosterone treatment to alleviate these problems. Men who use testosterone replacement therapy usually gain muscle mass and experience an emotional 'lift' and an increase in their libido.

Erectile dysfunction (impotence, or the inability to get or maintain an erection) can be caused by HIV damaging the nerves in the penis which control an erection (autonomic neuropathy). Similarly, anti-HIV drugs that cause neuropathy, such as ddC (zalcitabine, *Hivid*), ddI (didanosine, *Videx*) and d4T (stavudine, *Zerit*), may cause numbness in the genital area, which can make it difficult to sustain an erection. Protease inhibitors have also been reported to cause impotence, with some evidence suggesting that those containing ritonavir (*Norvir*) are particularly likely to cause sexual dysfinction.

Drugs including *Viagra* and *Cialis* are tablets used to treat impotence. They work by increasing blood flow to the penis, making it more sensitive to touch. However, these drugs should be taken with care by people using protease inhibitors, NNRTIs, ketoconazole, itraconazole or erythromycin. You should reduce by half the normal dose of the sexual dysfunction drug you are taking. For people taking ritonavir, it is recommended that *Viagra* should not be used at all, given the potential health risks. Similarly, the recreational drug poppers must not be used with *Viagra* or *Cialis*.

Further reading

NAM factsheets, *Candida, Chlamydia, Condoms, Gonorrhoea, Genital warts, Hepatitis B, Hepatitis C, Infectiousness, Herpes, Mother-to-baby transmission, Oral sex, Post-exposure prophylaxis, Pregnancy and conception, Primary infection, Pubic lice and scabies, Sexual dysfunction, Sperm washing, Syphilis, Sexual health check-ups* and *Unprotected sex.*

HIV and hepatitis, HIV and sex and *HIV and women,* booklets in the information for HIV-positive people series produced by NAM.

'Safer sex' in NAM's *AIDS Reference Manual* (last updated in June 2003).

Sexually transmitted infections: a guide for people with HIV, leaflet produced by the Terrence Higgins Trust.

My experience of anal warts

I've had warts since I was a child – they run in my family. At one point, around the age of 12, I had small warts on most of my fingers. Although I never sought treatment, after a year they suddenly disappeared within the space of a week.

My first bout of genital warts was similarly uneventful. I came home from my first year at university with a self-diagnosis of piles – an unbearable itch in my back passage, and pain and blood after using the toilet. I came away from the GP with an instruction to visit a 'treatment centre' 20 miles away. After being quizzed about my sexual history, an examination revealed the presence of an anal fissure and a single anal wart. The wart was quickly dispatched with a blast of liquid nitrogen.

Eight years later, a couple of years after my HIV diagnosis, the warts on my fingers, plus a few tiny ones on my chin, had returned and been removed with a quick nitrogen zap. When a subsequent examination revealed the presence of a few warts around my back passage, I assumed that a few icy blasts would see them off.

I diligently followed my doctor's advice to pop into the clinic a couple of times a week to have the warts sprayed. I was encouraged by the nurses' reassurances that the warts were small and would soon be gone – especially as my viral load had plummeted from over 120,000 to below 50 copies/ml within a month of starting therapy.

As my bi-weekly visits started to stretch over weeks, then months, a trip back to my doctor revealed that the three months of cryotherapy had achieved nothing, probably on account of my sluggish CD4 count response – rather than climbing obediently, it had continued to fall before hovering around 130 for most of my first year on therapy.

In the two-month wait to be seen by a surgeon, the warts, no longer being kept in check by their regular cold shower or by imiquimod cream, grew to grotesque proportions. One grew inside my anal canal and prolapsed every time I used the toilet, eventually becoming more than 5cm in length and unbelievably painful. I felt disgusting and my sex drive evaporated.

I pinned my hopes on the operation. However, nothing (and no-one) had prepared me for how painful this would turn out to be. After three days in hospital on intravenous antibiotics, there followed eight weeks of a degree of pain I had never imagined. I became terrified of using the toilet, necking laxatives and painkillers in handfuls and teetering on the edge of depression.

To top this off, the warts returned, even stronger, within a month of the surgery. On a return to see the surgeon, he nonchalantly informed me he "would have to repeat the procedure". Gritting my teeth through another three-month delay on a waiting list, the warts became larger than ever: I could barely walk for hours after using the toilet, and I was in tears most days.

Luckily, the second operation was far less traumatic than the first. I was up and ready to leave within hours of coming round, and felt better within days. I only had moderate pain for around a week.

In the two months since the procedure, there is no sign of a recurrence, although the few small warts that couldn't be excised are now enjoying their weekly nitrogen fix. Despite a diagnosis of grade I anal intraepithelial neoplasia (AIN), which is now being monitored in a clinical trial, my mood is climbing almost as quickly as my CD4 count. I'm back on my bike, and finally, after over a year, I'm no longer scared of the toilet.

Hard times, by Ben

For years I've been unable to get an erection.

I should be able to at my age, I'm only 34. But I just can't. When I'm having sex it just gets a bit harder – well, for a short time at least – before shrivelling back to normal size.

I used to think that the cause was all in my mind, but was forced to dismiss this when it became clear that I couldn't even get hard enough to masturbate.

Nor is illness the cause. To be honest, I've hardly had a day of illness since I was diagnosed with HIV six years ago.

It seems that it's a side-effect of the anti-HIV treatment I've been taking for about five years.

Okay, it's not the worst side-effect in the world, but it really has made me feel down. My self-confidence has really suffered.

It took a lot of courage to tell my doctor that I couldn't get an erection. To be honest, I felt a bit ashamed. I also thought that as HIV is sexually transmitted, my inability to get an erection was not something that would greatly concern the staff at my HIV clinic.

But it was taken seriously. My doctor didn't bat an eyelid and appeared to be concerned for me, particularly when I told him I'd been having problems for years, and referred me to one of his colleagues. I was prescribed *Viagra*. Although I'd heard it was a wonder drug, I had no great expectations, and was surprised and pleased in equal measure when I found that it worked.

Not only does it mean that I can get an erection again for the first time in years, but my self-confidence has returned and my general mental health improved.

Because I can be sure of getting, and staying, hard, I'm really confident using condoms.

I'm glad that I admitted to myself that I had a problem. There was an easy solution which has really improved the quality of my life.

Mother-to-baby transmission of HIV

Introduction

An HIV-positive woman can pass on HIV to her baby during pregnancy, or during delivery, or by breast-feeding.

Anti-HIV treatment can, however, greatly reduce the risks of a woman passing on HIV to her baby. Having a caesarean rather than a vaginal delivery can reduce the risks even further. The exclusive use of formula feed is strongly recommended for all babies with HIV-positive mothers in the UK. Using these methods, it's possible to reduce the risk of mother-to-baby transmission of HIV from about one in four to less than one in a hundred.

A number of factors can make it more likely that a woman will pass on HIV to her baby. These include:

- Being ill because of HIV.

- Having a high HIV viral load and a low CD4 cell count.

- Waters breaking four hours or more before delivery.

- Having an untreated sexually transmitted infection at the time of delivery.

- Using recreational drugs, particularly injected drugs, during pregnancy.

- Having a vaginal delivery (rather than a caesarean delivery) if HIV viral load is detectable.

- Having a difficult delivery, requiring, for example the use of forceps.

- Breastfeeding.

Preventing mother-to-baby transmission with anti-HIV drugs

Introduction

Taking anti-HIV drugs can dramatically reduce the risk of you passing on HIV to your baby. There are two different ways in which these drugs act.

First, they reduce your viral load so your baby is exposed to less HIV while in the womb and during birth. The aim of HIV treatment is to get, and keep, your viral load below 50. This is often referred to as an undetectable viral load.

Second, anti-HIV drugs may cross the placenta and enter your baby's body, preventing the virus from ever taking hold. Newborn babies are given a short course of anti-HIV drugs after they are born when their mother is known to be HIV-positive.

Two drugs have been shown to be very effective at preventing mother-to-baby transmission of HIV in the second of these ways. These are the nucleoside analogue (NRTI) AZT (zidovudine, *Retrovir*) and the non-nucleoside (NNRTI) nevirapine (*Viramune*). It's also likely that other drugs are also very effective, but these haven't been tested as extensively.

The ways in which anti-HIV drugs are used (on their own or in combination with other anti-HIV drugs) will depend on the damage HIV has done to your immune system, and the point in your pregnancy when your HIV was diagnosed.

In the UK, and other countries where there is easy access to anti-HIV drugs, nevirapine should not be used by itself (as monotherapy) to prevent mother-to-baby transmission of HIV, because resistance to the drug can rapidly develop if it is used in this way. Using it alone would limit your ability to benefit from nevirapine or related drugs in the future, when you may need them to protect your own health. Nor should nevirapine be used in combination with other HIV drugs if you have a CD4 cell count above 250, as there is a risk of potentially dangerous side-effects.

In good health?

If you have a CD4 cell count that is high enough to protect you from becoming ill because of HIV, and a low HIV viral load, and you are not ill because of HIV, then UK doctors recommend that you should receive treatment with AZT during the final three months (third trimester) of pregnancy. You will also be given an intravenous dose of AZT during labour, and will need to have a caesarean rather than a vaginal delivery.

Another option is to take a short course of three anti-HIV drugs during the last few months of pregnancy in order to get your viral load below 50. You will then have the option of having a planned vaginal delivery.

Your baby will need to take AZT syrup for four to six weeks.

High viral load, low CD4 cell count?

If HIV has damaged your immune system, meaning that you are vulnerable to infections, or if you have a high viral load, then you are advised to take three anti-HIV drugs, including the NRTIs AZT and 3TC, the NNRTI nevirapine or a protease inhibitor. You should not take nevirapine if your CD4 cell count is above 250. The higher your viral load, the earlier in pregnancy you will need to start taking treatment. If your viral load is still above 50 before delivery, then you will need to have a caesarean delivery. However, a viral load below 50 should mean that you have the option of a planned vaginal delivery.

Your baby will need to take four to six weeks of AZT syrup.

Already on treatment?

If you become pregnant whilst taking anti-HIV drugs that are successfully suppressing your viral load, you are recommended to continue taking them. You will need to have a special scan at week 20 of your pregnancy, called an anomaly scan, to see if your baby is developing with abnormalities.

Your baby will need to take four to six weeks of AZT syrup.

Diagnosed late in pregnancy?

If you are diagnosed with HIV very late during pregnancy (week 32 or later), then you will need to start taking a combination of three anti-HIV drugs immediately. These should be AZT, 3TC and nevirapine (unless your CD4 cell count is above 250, in which case nevirapine should be replaced with a protease inhibitor). These drugs are able to rapidly pass across the placenta into your baby.

Your baby will need to take four to six weeks of AZT syrup.

Diagnosed during delivery or afterwards?

If you find out you have HIV during delivery, or just after, then you should be given a dose of AZT by injection and oral doses of AZT and nevirapine. Your baby will also need to take a triple combination of anti-HIV drugs.

Safety of treatment to prevent mother-to-baby transmission of HIV

There's some evidence that there's a slightly increased risk of having a premature or low birth-weight baby if a mother takes anti-HIV drugs, particularly a protease inhibitor, during pregnancy. However, this is a controversial issue and there's also evidence showing that protease inhibitors do not cause premature birth.

Preventing mother-to-baby transmission of HIV – delivery

The risk of you passing on HIV to your baby is reduced if it is delivered using a planned surgical delivery. This is called an 'elective caesarean' and is scheduled to take place in the 38th week of pregnancy, but will be performed sooner if labour begins early. Taking anti-HIV drugs during a caesarean delivery reduces the risk of you passing on HIV to your baby to very low levels. However, as with all surgery, a caesarean delivery carries some risk, and these should be fully discussed with you before you give your consent to the procedure.

You are strongly recommended to have a caesarean if you have a detectable viral load, or if the only anti-HIV drug you took during pregnancy was AZT.

If your viral load has been consistently undetectable during pregnancy then you should be able to have a managed vaginal birth. This means that your doctors and midwife will make sure that your labour doesn't last too long and will take action to reduce the risk of you passing on HIV to your baby.

Preventing mother-to-baby transmission of HIV – infant feeding

The risk of you passing on HIV to your baby by breastfeeding can be as high as one in eight. In the UK and other countries where safe alternatives to breastfeeding are available, you are strongly recommended to feed your baby using formula feed from birth. Detailed advice and support on how to do this is available from your medical services and you should ask for help if you have difficulties meeting the cost.

Further reading

NAM factsheets, *Mother-to-baby transmission*, *Pregnancy and conception*, and *Sperm washing*

Anti-HIV drugs, HIV and children, HIV and women, and *HIV therapy* booklets in the information for HIV-positive people series produced by NAM.

'HIV transmission' in NAM's *AIDS Reference Manual* (last updated in June 2003).

Starting a family leaflet produced by the Terrence Higgins Trust.

Bun in the oven, by Susan Cole

I've gone and got myself knocked up. Got myself into trouble, bun in the oven, all the clichés of pregnancy that good Catholic (unmarried) girls should avoid. Pregnant and HIV-positive; a state that ten years ago would have been met with effusions of pity and foreboding. So how do I feel? Pretty good, actually.

I would love to take the moral high ground and claim that my pregnancy was planned with SAS precision and facilitated by a gleaming, sterile, turkey-baster. But I'd be lying. More like a one-off act of Easter abandon, probably brought on by the heady excess of too many chocolate eggs. I suppose I could be held up as a harsh example to teenage girls in convent school – you only need to do it once to get pregnant. Okay, I may have done the deed many more times than once, but it was the one unprotected time and BANG, up the duff. Not bad for a 35-year-old with geriatric ovaries hurtling towards menopause.

I found out I was enceinte in Geneva, attending a conference. I did a wee on the pregnancy stick in my hotel room, expecting the result to be negative, but a faint blue line on the stick appeared, screaming: "You've got a bun in the oven, Girlfriend!"

Reeling, I picked up the phone and called the first person who came to mind at midnight – my HIV doctor. He was wonderfully reassuring and congratulatory, despite his patient from Hell calling hysterically in the middle of the night. He reassured me that the risk of transmission to the baby was less than 1% as I had an undetectable viral load and, more surprisingly, that I did not need to change my medication. My blind panic gradually changed into pleasure (with just the tiniest hint of fear).

My partner was initially paralysed with shock but has become rather pleasantly supportive and even turns a blind eye to my slovenly slothfulness.

The first few months of pregnancy haven't been too bad. I haven't been sick, despite the fact that in my previous two pregnancies I chucked up for England every day. I have been feeling exhausted and have fallen asleep a couple of times at my desk. Mild pregnancy stress-incontinence doesn't go so well with the hay fever season and sneezing all day, but at least it's encouraging me to do my pelvic floor exercises.

I kept my pregnancy very quiet until I had my twelve-week scan. I was terrified that the my medication would lead to some gross deformity in the baby. It was wonderful seeing all its bits in order. I can't decide whether to have a caesarean or a vaginal delivery and I still worry about the tiny chance that the baby will have HIV.

Everyone has been very supportive about the news.

This first appeared in the September 2004 edition of Positive Nation magazine.

Matilda

I found out about my HIV status when I was 16 weeks pregnant. After I had an HIV test, I had counselling with the midwife. I told her of feeling utter disbelief about my situation and fear of how I was going to break the news to my partner. Yet, when I finally told my partner, he turned out to be understanding and supportive. I also encouraged him to take an HIV test, and he agreed, and fortunately he was negative. Since that time we have practiced safe sex.

At the same time, I told my HIV doctor and my midwife that I accepted their advice to start on early HIV treatment because I wanted to minimise the risk of infecting my unborn baby. The midwife told me that it is best if you don't breastfeed and that if you want you can have a caesarean section. I agreed with this, as by doing so you can greatly reduce the risk of infecting the baby. I also told my HIV doctor that I wanted my baby, when it was born, to take the anti-HIV medicine, AZT. Fortunately, I had a very healthy baby at the end.

I think that it is very important for pregnant African women to take an HIV test and if found positive, to start early treatment and accept other medical interventions which can help protect your unborn baby from HIV. My little girl is now four and half years old and she is negative. Thank God for that.

This testimony was first published on the Positvely Women website. Thanks to the author and Positvely Women for giving permission to reprint it here.

Mental health

Introduction

Mental health problems can affect anybody, but it seems that people with HIV are more likely to experience a range of mental health problems, not least because the groups most affected by HIV in the UK, gay men, refugees and migrants and drug users, are already more likely to have mental health problems. Advanced HIV infection itself is known to cause mental health problems, although these are now very rare. More common are feelings of acute emotional distress which often accompany adverse life-events and clinical mental disorders such as depression and anxiety. In addition, some anti-HIV drugs can cause psychological disturbance.

HIV-related mental disorders

It is estimated that before anti-HIV treatments became widely used, 7% of people with advanced HIV infection would develop dementia. Mania has also been observed in people with advanced HIV disease. It is highly unusual for a person who has been treated with anti-HIV drugs to develop either of these conditions as a direct result of being HIV-positive.

Symptoms of dementia include:

• Difficulty in thinking or understanding, such as forgetfulness, loss of memory, loss of concentration and confusion.

• Changes in behaviour, including loss of interest, feelings of isolation and childishness.

- Problems with movement and coordination, such as loss of balance or strength from the limbs.

There can be many causes of the symptoms listed above, including depression and infections, as well as dementia. So, it's very important to see your doctor to find out what the real cause is.

Some anti-HIV drugs appear to offer protection against the development of dementia. The first anti-HIV drug seen to help prevent dementia developing and as a treatment for the condition was AZT (zidovudine, *Retrovir*). More recently, d4T (stavudine, *Zerit*) and abacavir (*Ziagen*) have also been shown to offer protection against dementia and to help prevent the condition. A study has also suggested that combinations containing efavirenz (*Sustiva*) may be effective.

The reason why only some of the currently available anti-HIV drugs work against dementia is because the brain and spine are separated from the blood by the blood-brain barrier, which only allows very small molecules to get into the central nervous system. AZT, d4T, abacavir and efavirenz's (*Sustiva*) effects on dementia are thought to be due to their ability to cross the blood-brain barrier, achieve effective levels and fight HIV in the brain. Some researchers argue that any anti-HIV regimen that significantly improves the immune system should also improve dementia, as immune cells can cross the blood-brain barrier.

Emotional distress

Particular events such as receiving an HIV diagnosis, bereavement, the break down of a relationship, financial worries or work problems, or dealing with side-effects of treatment can result in feelings of deep unhappiness and emotional distress which are difficult to manage and interfere with a person's ability to get on with daily life.

Support from family and friends can be very helpful at these times, as can professional help, such as helplines and counselling. Many HIV clinics have specialist mental health teams and some HIV support agencies can offer short courses of counselling.

Some people also find that complementary therapies, such as acupuncture, can relieve some of the symptoms of emotional distress, although these are now rarely provided by HIV clinics.

Depression

Depression is a clinical illness and is twice as common in people with HIV as in the general population.

Depression can be triggered by illness or social problems, but it is not uncommon for there to be no readily identifiable cause. It is characterised by the presence of most or all of the following symptoms on a daily basis for several weeks: low mood; apathy; poor concentration; irritability; insomnia; early waking or oversleeping; inability to relax; weight gain or weight loss; loss of pleasure in usual activities; feelings of low self-worth; excessive guilt; and recurrent thoughts of death or suicide.

If you are diagnosed with depression, your doctor may recommend that you take antidepressant drugs, which relieve the symptoms of depression by altering chemicals in the brain which influence mood and behaviour. They can take several weeks to work and may have side-effects.

Although there are three classes of antidepressant drugs used (tricyclics; MAOIs; and SSRIs), it is most likely that you will be offered a drug from the SSRI (selective serotonin re-uptake inhibitors) class, which includes drugs like fluoxetine (*Prozac*), as these have fewest side-effects and interactions with other drugs. It is not uncommon for drugs in this class to cause sexual problems. You must not take the herbal antidepressant St John's wort if you are taking a protease inhibitor or an NNRTI.

The amount of time you stay on antidepressants will depend on your individual circumstances, and although you may start to feel better soon after starting to take them, it is recommended that you remain on them for at least three months if it is your first depressive illness, or longer if your depression has recurred.

Mental health problems as a side-effect of anti-HIV treatment

It is known that the anti-HIV drug efavirenz (*Sustiva*) can cause psychological disturbances. Some people have difficulty sleeping, or vivid dreams or nightmares. Other people have reported depression without any other apparent cause.

Anxiety

Anxiety is a feeling of panic or apprehension, which is often accompanied by physical symptoms such as sweating, rapid heart beat, agitation, nervousness, headaches and panic attacks. Anxiety can accompany depression or be seen as a disorder by itself, often caused by circumstances which result in fear, uncertainty or insecurity.

If anxiety is caused by practical problems, then getting advice, talking the problem through or counselling might be helpful. Anxiety which accompanies depression is relieved by antidepressant drugs. Some people find massage or other complementary therapies help relieve the symptoms of anxiety.

Drugs such as benzodiazepines, including valium, are now very rarely prescribed as a treatment for long-term anxiety because they are addictive. However, they are still used in the treatment of short periods of acute anxiety without any long-term dependency problems.

Talking therapies

Often drug therapies for mental problems work better if accompanied by talking therapies designed to help people understand and control their feelings. Examples include psychotherapy and cognitive behavioural therapy (CBT), both of which usually involve a short course of sessions with a psychotherapist or psychologist.

Further reading

NAM factsheets, *Dementia* and *Mental health*.

Adherence and *Anti-HIV drugs*, booklets in the information for HIV-positive people series produced by NAM.

'Symptoms and illnesses' in NAM's *HIV and AIDS Treatments Directory*.

Depression leaflet produced by the Terrence Higgins Trust.

Coping, by Frank

I started to write about my experiences of learning to cope with HIV some time ago. The unpleasant memories it forced me to recall upset me so much I had to take a break.

I was diagnosed with HIV in March 1991 after several months of ongoing severe flu-like symptoms. HIV wasn't much spoken of then and I wasn't really aware of it. Nor did I really think that I was at any real risk.

For the past year I'd been in a relationship which had recently ended after months of violence – included forced sex. My partner had not told me that he was HIV-positive and I'd not picked up on any clues to suggest that he might have HIV.

The disappointment and frustration of the relationship break-up had left me emotionally exhausted and physically weak. It was only some months later that I considered the possibility of HIV and asked my doctor for an HIV test, which was positive.

The consultant I was referred to was very supportive, and gave me time to ask questions. I pressed him for an indication of my prognosis, and he said that I could probably expect to live for another two years.

On the basis of this information, I made a will, distributed most of what I owned to family and others – and waited.

Fortunately I had some very good friends who I could confide in, and talking things over with them was the single greatest support I had during those awful months. It was a great relief just to be with them doing simple things, comfortable that they knew and understood me and what I was going through.

Gradually, I got stronger and was able to resume living a life and socializing. I began to enjoy each day as it came. I read a lot, and went away for holidays. I socialised with friends who understood my situation.

My friends knowing that I had HIV made a great difference. It meant that I could opt out of arrangements, leave dinner parties early, and, when I was on holiday, rest without people being offended. I could also take my medicines without explanation or embarrassment. That's not to say I was a total bore – I did make an effort.

There were still some bad times when medicines caused serious side-effects. I tried to remove stress from my life by lightening my work-load and responsibilities.

There was also a void in my life – a lack of physical and emotional intimacy. For five years I was celibate.

Then, nine years after my diagnosis, I met my partner, Michael, and we have been very happy ever since. It helped that he knew my status from the start. We met with my consultant together and discussed my health. I believe firmly that his support and understanding, his affection and love have been the main factor in my well-being. His very interest in my health and well-being has been life-enhancing for me.

The medical staff, my family, friends and partner have each played their own invaluable, unique and greatly appreciated part in my survival for so long with HIV, and have wonderfully enriched my life.

Depression, by Jonnie

I've never had a physical illness which I could say was really caused by HIV. But I have had terrible mental health problems, and although I'm sure there have been a lot of factors involved, I've no doubt that having HIV has contributed to the bouts of depression I've had in recent years.

Looking back, I can see that I've had occasional episodes of depression since my late teens, but it wasn't until a few years ago, after I'd had HIV for three years, that I became really unwell with depression.

I'd stopped work soon after I was diagnosed with HIV and went onto quite good state benefits. I had enough money to live on and kept myself more or less busy seeing friends, going to the gym, and sleeping off the night before. I felt more or less okay, with just the odd bored hour here or there to fill.

After a year or so of this, I noticed a few subtle changes. The occasional bleak moods lasting a few weeks seemed to be occurring more frequently and to be becoming more severe. What's more, I was starting to feel isolated, and thought that I was losing my social skills.

I've never been the deepest sleeper, but I noticed that I was finding it harder to drop off and waking early. Although I was tired all the time, I could never relax. I even started to avoid doing things which I used to enjoy – everything became a chore. This led to me thinking "what's the point?" Frighteningly, the answer I came up with was "there isn't one". Increasingly I started to think that death was desirable, and even began to think about suicide.

I even started to plan how I was going to do it and told myself it was no great loss – after all, I was going to die of AIDS anyway.

I knew I needed help and mentioned that I felt "a bit" depressed at my next appointment with my HIV doctor. I thought he'd recommend counselling and tell me to pull myself together. However, he immediately prescribed some antidepressants and referred me to see a specialist HIV psychiatrist.

My mood got better a few weeks after I started the antidepressants, and by the time my appointment with the psychiatrist came around I told myself I was better and didn't need it. Anyway, wasn't it only mad people who went to see psychiatrists? Nevertheless I went along and was told I had had a major depression. As well as taking antidepressants for about nine months, I had some talking therapy called cognitive behavioural therapy, which was designed to help me to understand why I got depressed and how to cope with it.

I realised a lot of things were contributing to my depression. Although I always told my friends I was cool about having HIV, I realised it really affected me. As had my childhood and growing up gay. I also came to see that the way I'd handled my HIV diagnosis wasn't helping either and that I was isolating myself. To help remedy this, I went to college part-time, then did some voluntary work before getting a part-time and then a full-time job.

I've had bleak moments since this and had to take another course of antidepressants, but things haven't been as bad as they were, partly because I accepted that I have to take my mental health as seriously as my physical health.

Russ

It is about nine years since I was told I was HIV-positive and it is almost the same amount of time since I met my partner, Chris, and started a stable relationship. These statements seem to run in tandem but the paths between them have been anything but smooth. My story is about denial, emotional feelings and the role that HIV can play in the creation and development of personal relationships. It is, in short, a truthful account of the emotional difficulties I have encountered – which you may have empathy with.

My partner Chris is HIV-negative and has been well throughout the whole period, but I must go back to the start of August 1995 to begin my story.

Being HIV-positive and single seemed natural. This hidden, awful virus did not exactly make me feel good about myself. The doctors were telling me I had only a few years to live, so somehow the idea of searching for a partner seemed futile. If I had only a short time to live, I certainly did not see any benefit in using up time and energy on emotional issues. Instead, I went out drinking nearly every night, and slept around, worked hard, socialised a lot and tried to enjoy every minute of the day. I remember feeling very tired, but put that down to HIV, and not my lifestyle. When illness came, I would enlist the support of members of the caring professions. Single, free, happy and busy, with a back-up. I really thought I had it all worked out. Maybe you have felt that, or perhaps you feel it now, and there is no doubt it is a nice feeling. Then one evening, at the start of one of my drinking binges, I met Chris. I was buzzing and felt confident and happy. One of the first things he said to me was that I had sad eyes. In one second, my whole life seemed to stop in the face of such directness. I felt the need to retaliate, and told him I was HIV-positive very much in the vein of "take that". The response? A kiss of passion and the word "So?"

So Chris entered my life when I did not want anyone. For me, facing up to HIV meant addressing the emotional as well as the medical issues. In short, it was permissible for me to love someone and even more important for someone to love me. Some of you will be laughing or sneering about this, perhaps — but remember at the time I am talking about, 1995, the life expectancy of most people living with HIV was quite short.

Now I was starting to feel emotions and that should have been good, but it did not work that way. I felt sad, hopeless and anxious, and furthermore I felt lonely. How could I be lonely when I was living with my partner? Then I felt envious of his good health and thought about how I had once been. A few years into the relationship, I was a mess and was being treated for depression. You see, this is no

Hollywood love story. The recovery does come, or else I would not be writing this, but it was difficult. It involved long-term counseling and a hell of a lot of effort on the part of Chris and myself. In short, I learned to involve myself in Chris's life and found my self-identity again as Russ, not Russ who is HIV-positive.

Coping with illness, going into hospital, end of life issues

Coping with illness

Introduction

Despite anti-HIV treatments, people with HIV in this country still experience illness. There are about 500 new AIDS diagnoses every year in the UK, and 400 AIDS deaths. This chapter looks at some of the practical things that can be done to make your life easier if you are experiencing illness because of HIV.

In many cases, it will be possible to successfully treat your illness and you'll return to full health. Or it may be that you experience a side-effect, caused by a medicine you are taking, which either goes away or lessens in its severity with time.

However, if you have a very weak immune system and you lose strength, illnesses can become more persistent and harder to fight off, meaning that you need long-term help coping with the effects of illness.

Living an independent life at home can become harder in these circumstances, but there are ways in which you can be assisted to do this. Your local council will have a social services department which will be able to offer a wide range of social care in your own home. Local voluntary organisations can also be helpful offering advice and practical and emotional support. What's available will depend on where you live, and it's important to remember that many local HIV organisations have closed or merged in recent years or have redirected their services towards other areas.

Often, however, it's partners, family, friends or other informal carers who provide the most important support. Informal carers can be put under a lot of practical and emotional strain. They have their own responsibilities to consider, as well as caring for you, and caring for somebody who is ill will inevitably have an emotional impact on them.

The following are key professionals who may provide important services that will allow you to maintain your independence at home during periods of illness.

GPs and primary care

GPs are the only doctors who can visit you in your home. They can also arrange for other health professionals to come to your home, including community nurses. Some hospitals have specialist teams that act as a link between the hospital where you receive your care and local community health services. They can put you into contact with GP and community health services, and sometimes provide direct care themselves.

Community nurses

Community nurses can provide support, help and advice with all the practical aspects of coping with illness and taking medication at home, including changing dressings, looking after an intravenous drip, and taking/giving injections.

They can teach you, or the people looking after you, how to take or give medicines by drip or injection and how to manage some of the problems of illness, such as lifting and bathing. Some community nurses also have specialist skills, for example pain control.

Occupational therapists

Occupational therapists (who are based both in hospitals and in council social services) offer practical ways of improving your quality of life, based on an understanding of your physical and emotional needs and your home environment.

After an assessment involving a detailed discussion of your needs and problems, an occupational therapist will try and work out with you how to solve practical problems at home, how to make tasks easier for you, and how to adapt your home to make it easier to live in and get around.

Palliative care

Palliative care aims to control symptoms and pain and improve quality of life. Palliative care aims to reduce the discomfort and pain of illness (or, indeed treatment side-effects) to a minimum. Some HIV clinics have doctors who are specialists in palliative care or pain control, and there are also nurses, physiotherapists, occupational therapists, dietitians and other members of your healthcare team who can also help.

Going into hospital

Introduction

There may be times when you need to be admitted to hospital, either to receive a course of treatment for an infection, for surgery, or even to participate in a clinical trial. For most people, going into hospital will be an unsettling, even frightening experience.

When you are first admitted, a nurse will fill out an admission form with you. This will record your name, address, date of birth, next of kin, and religion. You'll also be asked to provide a medical history and say how able you are to look after yourself. If you are having an operation, you'll be asked to give your consent. What an operation involves and why it's being undertaken should be fully explained to you before you give your consent. If anything is unclear, make sure you ask for more information.

Hospital routines can seem very strange. You might find that you have to get up and eat your meals earlier than you are used to doing. You may also feel like you have very little privacy or time to yourself. Ward rounds, medication rounds, consultations with doctors and tests can all feel overwhelming. On top of all this, you'll be away from loved ones and may also have to cope with bad news, illness, pain, or worries over an operation.

You may well see a number of different doctors whilst you're in hospital, and there's a chance that your regular HIV doctor won't be one of them. This can make it harder to ask questions about your treatment and care. If you don't feel able to ask one of your doctors a question, try getting a nurse or other member of the healthcare team to act as an intermediary. Ward rounds, when a group of doctors go from patient to patient can be particularly intimidating. It can be distressing to hear your illness or health discussed as if you weren't there, or as if you were just an interesting problem. Don't be frightened to ask questions during a ward round or remind the doctors that you're there!

Large hospitals are also teaching centres and you may be asked if you can be examined by a medical student as part of their training. It's perfectly okay for you to say no if you are not happy to agree.

If you're admitted to hospital for a reason other than HIV, it would be a good idea to make sure that a doctor or nurse involved in your HIV care knows and liaises with the team providing your care whilst you are in hospital. This will ensure that you receive the right treatment and care.

Visitors

Visitors can really help you cope with a stay in hospital and, particularly on specialist HIV wards, you may find that you're allowed visitors at any time and not just during set visiting hours. But visits can be tiring, particularly if you are feeling unwell, or are weak after an operation or other medical procedure. If you don't feel up to visits, let your friends and family know. The nursing staff on the ward will support any decisions you make about visits.

You'll almost certainly find that hospitals treat same-sex and unmarried partners with respect. It's worth knowing that legislation introduced by the UK government in 2004 (but yet to be passed) will, for the first time, give the registered partners of gay people the legal right to visit their partner in hospital.

Making hospital more comfortable

Having some of your own possessions with you can make a stay in hospital a lot more comfortable and bearable. Some of the most important things you might want to have with you are toiletries, tooth brush and paste, a razor and shaving foam, some clothes to wear during the day, and something to entertain you such as books, magazines and a personal stereo player. Mobile phones can help keep you in touch, but there may be restrictions on their use on the ward. Having some cash will also probably be useful. Be careful with items of value or money as thefts from patients do occur in hospitals.

Hospital food is often the subject of jokes, and although real efforts have been made to improve it in recent years, you may find it unpalatable. It's okay for visitors to bring food in for you, or for you to order food to be delivered to you on the ward. If you're feeling well enough, you may even want to go out for a meal.

Confidentiality

Confidentiality can be an issue during your stay in hospital. It can be hard to conceal that you are HIV-positive if you are staying on a specialist HIV ward and you may want to restrict your visitors to people who already know that you have HIV. Hospital staff shouldn't reveal details about your diagnosis or care to anyone without your consent.

Discharge

You'll be discharged from hospital as soon as you're medically fit. In some circumstances, you may also be discharged into the care of another healthcare provider, such as a hospice.

Before you are discharged, the hospital should do the following:

- Make a follow-up appointment with the appropriate out-patient department. If you were admitted to hospital because of HIV-related causes, this will be at your HIV clinic.

- Give you a telephone number to contact in case of emergencies.

- Give you enough medication to last until your out-patient appointment.

- Ensure that you are able to cope with your medication at home, or that you have help to do so.

- Give you a letter, or discharge note, to give to your GP.

- Arrange for transport to get you home.

End of life issues

Introduction
Although the prognosis for people with HIV has improved dramatically since the advent of effective anti-HIV treatment, people still die because of HIV. There are some practical issues that you will need to consider if you are going to die. These include wills, sorting out your financial affairs, and even funeral choices.

Making a will
Even if you're in perfectly good health, it makes good sense to have a will. A will is the only way of making sure that your partner, family and friends inherit your property in the way you want. Make sure you get a solicitor's advice when drawing up your will. This will ensure that your will is valid. Although it's not advised, you can write your will on forms bought from stationers. Just make sure you appoint an executor (someone to look after your affairs), and that it's signed and witnessed in the presence of two people who won't benefit from the will.

Although the UK government has introduced legislation (which has yet to become law) to give the registered partners of gay people inheritance rights to property, until this becomes law gay partners (as well as unmarried partners, lovers and friends) have no right to inherit anything if there is no will, no matter how long a relationship may have lasted.

A 'living will'

This is a statement of what kind of medical help you would like to receive if you become seriously ill. It's also called an advanced care directive. It basically sets out what efforts you want doctors to make to try and keep you alive. It also makes clear who you want to make treatment decisions for you if you are unable to do so. A living will can be of great help to the people caring for you, should you ever get this sick.

Power of attorney

If you give someone 'power of attorney', they will be able to sign papers on your behalf when you are unable to do so. You need to see a solicitor to arrange this.

Property

The surviving spouse from a marriage (or a same-sex partner under the UK government's proposed civil partnerships legislation) will inherit a property you own should you die. If you are not married to your partner (or are gay, until the civil partnership legislation becomes law), you should specify that you want your partner to get your property in your will or change the ownership of your property to joint ownership. If you are renting a property with someone, you need to ensure that their name is on the lease along with yours.

Finances

When somebody dies, all their assets are frozen. This includes money in joint bank accounts. This can take some time to sort out after a death, so it's best to plan ahead and make sure that your partner is not dependent on a joint account for access to cash.

If you have a pension or life assurance policy, make sure that you've nominated the person you want to receive benefits from it after your death. If you haven't done this, the company will give the money to the closest living relative (whatever your will says).

If you have debts, remember that these will pass to your next-of-kin or main beneficiary in your will. If your debts are large, there are some circumstances when bankruptcy might be an option, particularly if you don't own your own home or have a lot of valuable possessions. Places like the Citizens Advice Bureau can tell you what's involved.

Funeral arrangements

If you want, you can arrange this before your death, or you can leave the arrangements to the executor you named in your will. If you haven't made a will, this will pass to your next of kin. New government legislation will recognise the registered partners of gay people as next of kin. You can say in your will what kind of funeral service you would like, and whether you'd like to be buried or cremated. Funerals can be very distressing occasions for partners, family and friends, and knowing what your wishes were can help make the event less stressful.

Further reading

NAM factsheets, *Prognosis*.

'Symptoms and illnesses' in NAM's *HIV and AIDS Treatments Directory*.

Billy

1980

When I first met Billy, I was working behind the bar at the Euston Tavern in Kings Cross. Billy had been staring across the bar at me for two months and I hadn't even noticed. Eventually his friends persuaded me to go to a party with them and we ended up standing together in the hall, talking for two hours. I finally realised what was going on – how naïve I was then, a 17-year-old law-breaker (in 1980 the age of consent for gay men was still 21).

1983

We got our first flat together with a borrowed settee, no bed and a fridge that arrived two weeks late.

Home furnishings were never important to Bill; we liked to travel: Barbados, Gambia, America. We saw the world.

1988

A black mark appeared on my leg, starting out as a bruise but turning completely black. It cleared, but if ever my leg scraped against anything these bruises kept appearing.

I visited my GP, who referred me to the local hospital. The consultant I saw suggested that I have a bone marrow test to check my platelet count. It was three.

Panic set in. The consultant seemed quite amazed that I was still breathing. She decided it was time for me to have the big test.

I gave the blood sample and was asked to return in a week. One week later, I was back in the waiting room where I sat. And sat.

Eventually my consultant arrived, looking extremely worried. She confirmed that I had thrombocytopenia, which

I already knew. I wanted to know the result of my HIV test.

It took her all her courage to tell me that she had lost the test result and that I would have to give more blood and wait another week. One week later, I had some more news: the blood had been sent somewhere else for "confirmation" and I would have to wait another week for the result.

Week three came and we had a result. To be honest, I really didn't care by then, having been messed around so much. I was positive.

I remember going home; Billy was in the bath and I sat on the toilet next to him and started crying. His only reply was, "thought so – don't worry." Not long after that Billy also tested HIV-positive.

1994

This was our big year: skiing in France, shopping in New York, partying in Ibiza, lots of weekends away.

Billy was feeling tired in July but still managed to visit the pub every night. He worked in the mornings and slept the afternoons away at home, unless it was sunny, when he would go sunbathing or take the dog to the park.

Trouble started in September, when Billy was made redundant. At the same time he started coughing, a cough that was to be persistent.

Our last holiday together was in Florida in November. Even though Billy was tired, we had a great time together: Disney, MGM, Universal. But on the flight back, Billy said he felt unwell and ended up spending most of the flight in the toilet, trying to cool down.

The first big bomb dropped about three days before Christmas. When we went to the pub together, standing face to face, he said to me, "I know I won't be here this time next year." It was the first negative thing he had said concerning his illness. I remember holding his head, putting it next to mine, and for a brief moment I knew he was telling the truth.

1995

Billy was off on holiday again in the Canaries, this time with a friend from work. I met them at the airport. As soon as I saw them walk through the arrivals door I started crying: Billy looked a shadow of himself (though still the beauty I knew).

In hospital the next day we were told that Billy had a collapsed lung and would have to stay in for a few days. He was determined to get out and go back to Ireland for another break, and told the staff he was going, collapsed lung or not.

Ireland wasn't to be: a filter was put on his lung but on the second day his other lung collapsed. In the course of the next month, both his lungs were operated on. Shortly after his second operation I got a call from a nurse, at 10pm. She said, "Billy can't come to the phone, but can you come up to the hospital now with two tubs of Haagen Daz ice cream?" He picked his moments.

Billy was in hospital for a long time, six weeks of which he was unable to move because of his filters, and we both felt the strain. I was tired, pissed off. I visited some mornings – went to work – back at lunch break – back to work – home to take the dog for a walk before going back to hospital and staying till late. Some nights we didn't even talk.

Although Billy was very frail and exhausted and his weight was down to seven stone, they allowed him home on 11th May.

Within five days, the home care team insisted he should go back to hospital. I dressed him and walked him to the car.

He was so thin that on the way to the car his trousers just came down. I was not ashamed.

On the way to the hospital I told him how much I loved him. This was something we always did, but this time I wanted to be sure he knew how much I meant it. He told me it had been a pleasure sharing his life with me. I drove to the hospital in tears.

At the hospital the doctors and nurses were ready for him and a private room had been prepared. Bells started ringing in my head and my body just crumbled; reality was setting in.

I rang a friend and my sister, Kay who, along with the rest of my family, had only known about Billy's illness for two weeks prior to this. Kay arrived and we held each other and cried.

Kay and I stayed on the bed next to Billy, though we didn't sleep. Billy woke twice, once to say he wanted to go home, and once to say he loved me. The morning took so long to arrive.

In the morning my mum arrived. It was so good to see her. Mum, Kay and myself just looked at each other and wept. Billy's sister and brother-in-law arrived in the afternoon, but they didn't want to know what was going on. His sister held Billy but his brother-in-law didn't know what to do.

I hadn't slept for ages, but at around 11.30pm I closed my eyes. I was woken at 12.35am to be told that Billy was going.

How can I ever explain in words how it feels to see someone you love slipping away? Anger, loneliness, emptiness. For the first time in our lives together there was nothing I could do. I remember smelling his hair, his breath, his being. But he was gone.

The care and love of the nurses on the ward was wonderful for Billy and for me and my friends. My friends were incredible and together they saw me through the lowest point of my life.

Until we meet again, Billy, I love you eternally.

Reprinted from the 1996 edition of Living with HIV and AIDS.

Going into hospital, by Christopher

My experiences of hospitalisation are mixed. I've been admitted twice in the last six months, both times for a minor operation. However, following the excellent standards of care I've received at my HIV clinic, I was surprised by my treatment as an in-patient on a general surgery ward.

Before my first operation, my care was exemplary. I attended a pre-surgical outpatient appointment, when I met the surgeon and was examined in preparation for the anaesthetic. On the day of the procedure, a steady stream of nurses, surgeons and anaesthetists visited me on the ward to take information, explain what was going to happen and give me the opportunity to ask any questions.

However, these standards were not maintained once I was back on the ward. It was clear that the nurses were too stretched to offer any care beyond rushing by the bed with the next paper cup of tablets. And as the day wore on, it became obvious that the surgeon was not planning to visit his patients to explain how their procedures had gone, or what to expect over the next few weeks – in my case, the worst pain I have ever experienced.

I was left feeling deeply frustrated. On top of that, I was only told at the last moment that I would have to remain on the ward for three days, rather than being able to go home that evening as promised.

Despite the lack of information, which I do not blame on the staff themselves but on the organisation of the hospital, I was pleasantly surprised by their attitude towards my HIV status (and low CD4 count) and daily visits from my gay partner – although the same could not be said for the other men in the ward, most of whom were over twice my age. I also found the hospital routine less dull than I had imagined – the meals were reasonable, if a little early, and I managed to catch up with some reading and complete a couple of newspaper crosswords. I even popped out for a few pints one evening, with the encouragement of the nurses.

But I came away with a deep resentment of the apparent lack of interest in my needs or wishes after my procedure. Although it is not in my nature, I made an active decision to make a fuss on my second admission, demanding the answers to questions about my treatment and care and questioning the doctors' decisions. This made the experience far more successful and satisfying. Nevertheless, I still left without the promised post-surgical visit from the surgeon, and even without the correct supply of drugs. I eventually saw the surgeon two months later, and was finally given some information about my procedure.

Complementary therapies

Reasons why people with HIV use complementary therapies

Introduction

Complementary therapies are used by a large number of people with HIV.

There's no consensus amongst HIV doctors about the role of complementary therapies in the treatment of HIV. Some doctors dismiss them out of hand, whilst others take a more open-minded view. This is partly because complementary therapies have not, on the whole, been subjected to the same rigorous assessment of their effectiveness and safety as licensed medicines.

Reasons for the use of complementary therapies include stress reduction, the relief of side-effects and symptoms, to relieve pain, and to boost the immune system.

Reducing stress

Many people use complementary therapies to reduce stress. They can also have added benefits, such as increasing a general sense of health and well-being.

Reducing treatment side-effects

The side-effects of HIV treatment, and of the drugs used to treat infections, can be improved by supplements and complementary medicines. For example, calcium supplements can help control diarrhoea, a very common side-effect of HIV treatment. Aromatherapy oils, such as rosemary and peppermint, can relieve feelings of nausea; and herbs, such as valerian, and relaxation therapies can help with disturbed sleep and anxiety.

Boosting the immune system

There's very little evidence, partly due to a lack of research, that complementary therapies can boost the immune system, despite the fact that this benefit is claimed for many treatments.

Slowing HIV disease progression

It's known that people with HIV often have certain nutritional deficiencies. This is a symptom of HIV infection rather than a cause of immune deficiency or opportunistic infections. Providing supplementation may help address these deficiencies, but there's very limited evidence that this will lead to any improvement in immune function or health.

Pain relief

Some forms of complementary therapy can provide effective pain relief. Acupuncture is commonly used to relieve pain, and massage therapies and osteopathy can also be effective, particularly for muscle or joint pain. Always tell your doctor if you experience anything other than mild pain, or if you are in persistent pain.

Treatment for infections

There's no evidence that complementary medicines can prevent or cure any major infection. You will be endangering your life if you choose an alternative approach for the treatment of a major infection such as pneumonia, which always requires appropriate antibiotic treatment. Having said that, herbal remedies, acupuncture and homeopaths can help relieve some of the symptoms of infections, such as night sweats.

Points to remember

Complementary therapies will not solve your health or life problems, so be realistic in your expectations of what they can deliver. For example, question whether your chosen therapy will help control your symptoms or side-effects, or simply make them easier to live with.

Complementary treatments don't have the same methods of rigorous regulation and control as conventional medicine. For this reason, treat with suspicion the claims made about the effectiveness of any therapy you are considering.

Just like conventional medicine, complementary therapies can have side-effects or can even be dangerous. What's more, herbal remedies can interact with anti-HIV drugs. For example, the herbal treatment for depression, St John's wort, can reduce levels of protease inhibitors and NNRTIs in the blood. Large doses of vitamin C can lower blood concentrations of the protease inhibitor indinavir, and large doses of garlic have been shown to reduce the level of the protease inhibitor saquinavir. Just because a treatment is "natural" doesn't mean that it's automatically safe or risk-free.

Choosing a therapist

Most complementary therapy practitioners will only see a few, if any, patients with HIV. It can therefore be hard to be confident that you are being treated by a practitioner who understands your situation. It's worth asking a few questions:

- What is the treatment you are offering and how can it benefit me? Different practitioners will approach the same therapy in different ways. If a practitioner makes amazing claims for the benefits of their therapy, such as an ability to cure HIV, they're best avoided, as is any practitioner who advises you to stop your anti-HIV treatment or other conventional treatment.

- What is your experience of treating people with HIV? It's important that your practitioner has a basic understanding of HIV. If they don't have this knowledge, they may miss important symptoms which you should bring to the attention of a doctor.

- What are your charges? Charges vary. Discuss and agree charges in advance. Be wary of any practitioner charging more than £60 for an initial assessment – the chances are that you're being overcharged. Many practitioners will have a sliding scale of fees depending on your income. Some HIV organisations offer some complementary therapies. These have been heavily cut back since effective anti-HIV treatments became available, so don't assume that a treatment you received for free in the past will still be available.

- What are your qualifications? Try and find out what qualification your practitioner has. This isn't necessarily a guarantee of competence or quality, as very few complementary therapies have the same rigorous regulation that governs conventional medicine.

Combining conventional and complementary therapies

Always tell your HIV doctor about any complementary therapies or supplements you may be using. Listen to any doubts your doctor might express about your chosen complementary approach. Although a good doctor will respect your choice, you should take note of any evidence he offers to show that a therapy doesn't have any benefit or is even harmful. On the other hand, if you have a major disagreement with your doctor it could be that another doctor at your HIV clinic has a more sympathetic attitude towards complementary therapies.

It's extremely important that you find out if you can combine your complementary therapies with your orthodox treatment. It's particularly important if you are taking herbal remedies or supplements of any kind. As mentioned before, some herbal remedies and supplements interact with anti-HIV drugs. As well as the interactions that are already known, there could well be others, as the way in which herbal remedies and medicines interact hasn't been studied very extensively.

You should tell your complementary therapist about any anti-HIV or other medicines you are receiving. This will help them to avoid interactions. Some complementary therapy practitioners take the view that orthodox medicines contribute to, or even cause, illness. They should, however, respect your choice to take conventional medicine.

It's always worth remembering that the dramatic improvements in the health of many people with HIV, and the fall in illness and deaths caused by HIV, are due to effective anti-HIV treatment. Treat with great suspicion any therapist who questions or denies this.

A-Z of complementary therapies

Introduction
The following is a very brief introduction to some of the complementary and alternative therapies used by people with HIV. A lot more information can be found in NAM's Directory of complementary therapies in HIV and AIDS, which is available free to people affected by HIV.

Acupuncture
This is an aspect of traditional Chinese medicine (see entry below). It involves the insertion of fine needles into different points of the body to improve the flow of energy. This is normally painless or involves only very mild discomfort. It can be helpful with coping with stress, fatigue and pain.

Aromatherapy
This uses essential oils extracted from plants. Each oil is supposed to have a different healing effect on the mind and body. They can be directly inhaled, or used in baths or massage. Aromatherapy is an effective treatment for stress and encourages relaxation. Some oils can be toxic, so it's worth seeing a qualified aromatherapist.

Autogenic training

This is a technique using daily mental exercises to reduce stress, directing the mind and body towards a state of deep relaxation and encouraging healing. It is credited with increasing energy and helping with sleeping problems. It may also help with certain symptoms such as breathlessness or night sweats.

Bach flower remedies

These are harmless, inexpensive remedies available from many wholefood shops. They are derived from wild flowers and claim a wide range of calming and restorative powers.

Dietary therapies

Diet plays a key role in many complementary and alternative therapies, but there are certain diets which claim to improve health and immunity. These include macrobiotic diets, anti-candida diets and organic, raw and whole food diets. All may have advantages, but changing your whole diet at once can be very difficult, and if you are ill, or have metabolic complications, it might not be a good idea at all. See a dietitian before making any major changes to your diet (for more see the chapter *Nutrition and HIV*).

Exercise

Any form of vigorous exercise will help improve your cardiovascular fitness, reduce your risk of heart disease, help you to maintain lean muscle mass, and improve your ability to fight infection (see the chapter *Exercise*). Exercise such as T'ai chi, yoga and the Alexander technique are disciplines which many find calm the body, mind and spirit.

Healing and therapeutic touch

There are many forms of healing through touch, including some based on faith and therapies such as Reiki. All seek to encourage healing through one person acting as a channel for energy to flow into another. Reported results include improvements in mental or physical health and greater relaxation.

Herbs

This is a form of medicine which uses plants or herbs to maintain health, treat illness and promote health. Herbal treatments can be used successfully to treat minor ailments, such as tea tree oil or garlic for some fungal infections. However, bad reactions can occur and herbal treatments can interact with medicines used to treat HIV. Always tell your doctor about any herbal therapy you are taking or thinking of taking.

Homoeopathy

In homoeopathy, tiny traces of a substance that would normally cause illness are used to treat the same illness. Symptoms are not repressed but encouraged as they are seen as the body's way of healing itself, and homoeopathic remedies are finely tuned to each individual. Homoeopaths approach HIV in different ways. Some aim to treat a particular infection or illness, other will be more concerned with damage to the immune system. Homoeopaths are as likely to be interested in your emotional symptoms as your physical symptoms.

Hypnotherapy

The trance-like state created by a hypnotist opens the mind to suggestion, which can help reduce symptoms and help with psychological treatment. It can help reduce stress and pain. However, it's vital that you use a reputable practitioner.

Massage

This is one of the simplest and most popular therapies. It is an excellent way of reducing stress and promoting a sense of well-being and can help relieve some of the side-effects of anti-HIV treatment.

Naturopathy

This is a drug-free healing process based on the principle that the body is able to heal itself, supported by changes in diet, fasting, sweating and exercise. However, naturopaths acknowledge the importance of medicines when they are needed, and focus their therapy in this instance on improving overall health and well-being.

Osteopathy

This is a physical, manipulative therapy which seeks to correct any structural dysfunctions in the body that are causing health problems. Recurrent chest pain, neck pain, problems with swallowing, breathing and bowel function can all be improved with osteopathy. It's widely used for muscle and joint pain, and can also improve general vitality.

Reflexology

Reflexologists treat the bottom of your feet as a map for your body, and by massaging specific areas of the feet seek to improve the health of the related part of the body. Reflexology can offer relief for specific symptoms and side-effects as well as reducing stress.

Shiatsu

This is a combination of massage and acupuncture, where pressure is applied to healing points on the body, improving the flow of blood and energy and increasing vitality. It's an effective treatment for stress, anxiety and related conditions such as insomnia. It can also be used to treat symptoms and side-effects such as nausea.

Traditional Chinese medicine

This is a medical discipline which uses concepts, language and methods which are completely different from medicine practiced in the west. It incorporates several different elements including qi gong, acupuncture (see above) and herbal remedies. Qi gong and acupuncture both focus on the balance of the energies, 'qi', in the body. Chinese herbal medicine has been practiced for thousands of years, and works by strengthening the immune system rather than by directly attacking an infection. Chinese herbal medicine can cause side-effects, and can also interact with prescription medication.

Visualisation

This uses mental imagery to fight illness and has been credited with an improvement in symptoms and an increase in energy levels.

Further reading

Anti-HIV drugs, HIV therapy, and *Nutrition,* booklets in the information for HIV-positive people series produced by NAM.

NAM's *Directory of Complementary Therapies in HIV and AIDS.*

'Drugs used by people with HIV' in NAM's *HIV and AIDS Treatments Directory.*

The Ikea approach

I've no doubt that the main reason that I'm alive and well after almost 14 years of living with HIV is because combination therapy became available in 1996, just as my immune system was starting to become so weak that I was vulnerable to AIDS-defining illnesses.

Well, eight years on, my T-cell count is over 1,000 and my viral load has been undetectable for years.

But as well as acknowledging how important HIV drugs have been, I also want to claim a bit of the credit for doing my bit to keep myself healthy and fit. It's what I call my "Ikea approach" (after the low-cost Swedish home furnishing store that keeps prices down by asking customers to collect their purchases from the warehouse, and assemble them themselves). Well, I met the medicines half-way by making sure I looked after myself.

First of all I make sure I take my anti-HIV pills. Okay, I've missed the odd dose, and taken some a few hours late. But I seem to have got away with it and am still taking my first combination (except for one change due to side-effects).

Then there's my diet. For the first few years after my HIV diagnosis I was obsessive about my diet, making sure that my diet, from my bowl of wholemeal porridge for breakfast, to my fruit salad desert after supper, was as healthy as possible. It may have been healthy, but it was also very worthy and, actually, boring. I'm now much more relaxed and more or less eat what I want, particularly as I once heard an HIV doctor say that being HIV-positive means "eating for two". Okay, I still make sure that I eat lots of fresh fruit and veg, and am easy on the lard, but now I allow myself food that I want to eat, not food that I feel I should eat.

I've always been pretty active and do a lot of exercise. Being honest, vanity was my main motivation to start off with – I found it was much easier to pull with a few muscles – but over the years, fitness and health has become more of a priority. I do a blend of weights and cardio and hope that's helped control my blood fats even though I'm taking a protease inhibitor.

At times I've used complementary and alternative treatments. For a few years, in the early 90s, I was actually quite into them. There seemed to be so little else I could do to fight HIV. I tried a few things, including acupuncture, high dose vitamins and Chinese herbs. Well, my T-cell count didn't go down when I was using them, but they still didn't prevent me getting a bad chest infection which meant a lengthy stay in hospital.

I do still use them though, but am realistic about what they can achieve. As far as I'm concerned, anti-HIV drugs are the reason I'm alive and well, the complementary stuff is just that – a desirable add-on, to help me feel more comfortable. Acupuncture helps me relax, and really did help to relieve the side-effects I experienced when I started my first combination. The odd massage makes me feel better, and I still take a multivitamin every morning. I figure it can't do me any harm, and might actually do me some good.

Having got my life back, I want to enjoy it. That hasn't always been easy. I've gone through some really bleak periods during the time I've had HIV and actually felt suicidal at times. Counselling helped at times, but at others talking about feeling bad and why I felt awful actually made things worse! Antidepressants helped a lot, though, as did some focused psychotherapy when I wasn't actually depressed.

Since I was a student, I've enjoyed a drink, and still do. I've also had some great times on drugs of various descriptions. Projectile vomiting and convulsing in a club after taking a pill a few months after starting HIV medicines was a bit of a wake-up call and I haven't touched anything since. I know a lot of people manage to mix medicines and recreationals, but that was just too frightening for me.

Just after my HIV diagnosis I bought a sofa from Ikea, thinking that as I wasn't going to last too long, it didn't matter if it didn't either. Well, the sofa, like me, is still here.

Money

Introduction

This chapter provides an introduction to some of the key issues involving money, welfare benefits and personal finance which you might encounter.

Money worries can be a real headache and often get worse if you don't take action, so it's important to tackle them as soon as possible. The information in this section isn't exhaustive, and if you are going to make a claim for welfare benefits, or are thinking of applying for a mortgage, you should seek specialist advice. Regulations governing access to benefits can change very quickly, so, even if you've made a successful application in the past, it's wise to get advice from an accredited benefits adviser. Similarly, some financial advisers have developed a detailed understanding of the financial issues faced by HIV-positive people. A good place to start if you want information on benefits or money advice is the Citizens Advice Bureau. Their website is www.citizensadvice.org.uk and they have branches around the country. All their advice is free.

State benefits

Incapacity benefit and Income Support

This section was written in late 2004. Rules regarding state benefits are continually changing. If you have any questions about state benefits you would be well advised to seek specialist advice.

If you are ill because of HIV and unable to work, you may be able to successfully apply for state welfare benefits.

There are two benefits which you can apply for if you are too ill to work: Incapacity Benefit and Income Support.

Incapacity Benefit is only paid to people who have made sufficient National Insurance contributions. It is not means tested, and you can receive Incapacity Benefit even if you are in receipt of a medical retirement pension.

Income Support is paid to people who are ineligible for Incapacity Benefit. It is a means tested benefit, which means that eligibility is assessed by looking at how much money you have coming in.

To claim either of these benefits you need to complete a claim form, which can either be downloaded from the internet from this website www.jobcentreplus.gov.uk or obtained from your local benefits office. You need to complete the claim form and send it back to your local benefits office, together with a medical certificate (often called a sick note) from your doctor saying that you are unfit for work. The medical certificate doesn't have to say that you are HIV-positive.

Your claim will then be assessed. As part of this, you will have what is called a Personal Capability Assessment, to see if you are able to undertake any form of work. As part of this assessment you may be asked to see a doctor, and the benefits officer might write to your HIV doctor to find out more about your health and ability to work.

If you are receiving Disability Living Allowance at the higher rate, you are exempted from the Personal Capability Assessment and will receive Incapacity Benefit or Income Support automatically.

After twelve months of receiving either Incapacity Benefit or Income Support because of illness, the amount of money you receive will automatically increase because you will be awarded an additional Disability Premium.

If you have been awarded a Disability Living Allowance care component at any rate, you will receive the Disability Premium from the moment you are awarded Incapacity Benefit or Income

Support. If you receive the medium or high rates of Disability Living Allowance care component you will also receive an additional disability premium.

If you are assessed as being able to work, you will need to apply for Job Seekers Allowance.

Disability Living Allowance

Disability Living Allowance (DLA) is paid in two components: one for care and one for mobility. The care component is paid at three levels: higher, medium, or lower, depending on the amount of care you need. The mobility component is paid in two components, a higher rate and a lower rate, depending on how much trouble you have getting around.

If you are very ill and could die within six months, you can make an application for the care component of DLA under the "Special Rules". You don't actually have to need any personal care for a special rules award, but in order to get it your doctor must complete a form providing a diagnosis.

If you are awarded the higher rate of the mobility component, you can use this to obtain a car on a lease arrangement through Motability.

DLA is a not means tested and nor is it taxed, and your eligibility to receive it is not dependent on the payment of National Insurance contributions.

Before anti-HIV treatments became available in the mid/late 1990s it was relatively easy for people with HIV to make a successful claim for DLA, often for an indefinite period. However, as people with HIV are now living longer and healthier lives, thanks to treatment, access to DLA has tightened up.

It is still possible for people with HIV to make successful claims for DLA, but the benefit is now mostly awarded for a set time period.

The DLA care components act as a trigger for the award of additional disability premiums, which you will receive on top of any Incapacity Benefit or Income Support you may be receiving.

It can be very daunting filling out forms which ask you detailed questions about your health. Specialist benefits advisors can offer information about making claims for benefits, and they can also look at your circumstances with you to see if you are eligible to claim any additional benefits, such as Child Benefit, Child Tax Credit, or the Disabled Person's Tax Credit.

Housing Benefit, Council Tax Credit

If you are receiving Income Support, you'll be eligible for help paying your rent and council tax. You may also be eligible for housing benefit and council tax credit if you are receiving Incapacity Benefit. You need to apply to your local council for these benefits. A benefits advisor will be able to provide you with information about making a claim.

Immigration status and access to benefits

People who are claiming asylum or leave to remain in the UK are not able to apply for any UK benefit.

Debt management

Organisations which provide benefits advice and information are often able to help you to work out how to manage any debts which you may have.

An advisor will look at your financial commitments and income with you. They'll prioritise your financial commitments and debts, giving the highest priority to your rent or mortgage, utility bills, council tax, and any fines which you may have. If you have any money left over, then a repayment scheme for credit cards, loans and other debts can be worked out. If you are very badly in debt, they will be able to advice you on bankruptcy or administration.

Even if you feel able to manage your own financial affairs, don't ignore letters from banks or credit card companies. Debts won't go away unless you do something about them, and will become more of a headache the longer you leave them.

Personal finance

It's an indication of how much the outlook for HIV-positive people has improved since effective treatment became available that this book includes a section providing information on mortgages and pensions.

Mortgages

Getting a mortgage is not actually any harder if you are HIV-positive. Mortgage lenders usually don't ask any questions about your health or HIV status. All they're interested in is seeing that you meet the financial criteria for the mortgage you are applying for.

However, there can still be problems. You may well be asked to take out life assurance to cover the mortgage in the event of your death. Even though the prognosis for many people with HIV has improved dramatically recently there's still no life assurance policy which will provide cover for people with HIV. Don't lie about your health to get life assurance cover. A better plan might be to find a mortgage lender that doesn't require life assurance.

It's also likely to be impossible for you to obtain heath insurance to cover your mortgage payments in the event of you becoming too ill to work. Again, don't lie. Your claim won't be successful and you'll just be wasting money on premiums.

Pensions

Having HIV will not be a problem if you are thinking of joining a company pension scheme or starting a personal pension plan. However, you might ask, why bother? Improving treatment for HIV could well mean that you live to pension age and beyond. What's more, if you were to become ill, or even die before retirement age, the terms of your pension could mean that you still get benefits from it, such as a medical retirement pension or, in the event of your death, a payment to your partner or next-of-kin.

It's worth getting specialist financial advice, and some financial advisers have a lot of experience of working with HIV-positive clients. Similar advice might also be available from your local HIV support organisation.

HIV and the law

by James Calmers

This section was written in late 2004. It was accurate at the time of going to print, but the law relating to HIV is subject to change, both because of rulings in the court and acts of Parliament. It's important to obtain specialist legal advice from a lawyer.

Confidentiality

Introduction

Confidential information may be protected by law. The House of Lords, the highest court in land, confirmed in 2004 that "a duty of confidence will arise whenever the party subject to the duty is in a situation where he knows or ought to know that the other person can reasonably expect his privacy to be respected."

But a ruling from 1990 puts some limitations on this:

• It only applies to information which is actually confidential. Once information enters the public domain, it is no longer protected by confidentiality.

• It does not apply to useless or trivial information.

• Although it is in the public interest that confidential information should be protected, that public interest may sometimes be outweighed by another public interest favouring disclosure. In such cases, the public interest in confidentiality must be balanced against the public interest in disclosure.

It is the third of these exceptions which is probably the most important in the context of HIV.

Confidentiality and HIV

As early as 1988 a case involving two doctors showed that HIV was covered by confidentiality. An unknown health authority employee (or employees) passed information regarding these doctors' HIV status to a newspaper reporter. The newspaper intended to publish an article identifying the doctors concerned and describing their condition. The health authority sought a court order preventing the newspaper from publishing the information, or using it in any other way, which was granted.

The court noted that there was a public interest in the freedom of the press, and also accepted that there was some public interest in the information which the newspaper sought to publish. However, "those public interests [were] substantially outweighed when measured against the public interests in relation to loyalty and confidentiality both generally and with particular reference to AIDS patients' hospital records."

Disclosure of confidential medical information in the public interest

Confidential medical information may sometimes be disclosed in the public interest. A ruling in 1990 involving a psychiatric patient confirmed that the public interest in protecting the safety of others outweighed the public interest in preserving an individual's right to confidentiality.

In certain circumstances, this principle may be relied upon to justify the disclosure of information about a person's HIV-positive status without their consent. The General Medical Council's Guidance to Doctors on Serious Communicable Diseases (1997) states as follows:

"You may disclose information about a patient, whether living or dead, in order to protect a person from risk of death or serious harm. For example, you may disclose information to a known sexual contact of a patient with HIV where you have reason to think that the patient has not informed that person, and cannot be persuaded to do so. In such circumstances you should tell the patient before you make the disclosure, and you must be prepared to justify a decision to disclose information. You must not disclose information to others, for example relatives, who have not been, and are not, at risk of infection."

The guidance also notes that confidential medical information may be disclosed to other health care workers if failure to disclose would put them at a serious risk of death or serious harm.

HIV transmission and the criminal law

Introduction

Up until relatively recently, it was thought that the transmission of HIV (at least through consensual sexual intercourse, or the sharing of drug-injecting equipment) could not amount to a criminal offence in the UK. In England and Wales, this was because the relevant offence – "unlawfully and maliciously inflicting grievous bodily harm" – had been interpreted by the courts in the nineteenth century as being restricted to cases where one person had attacked another, for example by striking a blow or using a knife. However, that interpretation of the offence changed over time, and it was gradually recognised that the offence could apply to any case of "causing" harm.

The first successful prosecution for HIV transmission in England and Wales was brought against Mohammed Dica, who was convicted of two counts of unlawfully and maliciously inflicting grievous bodily harm in October 2003. Although his conviction was later quashed by the Court of Appeal (because the judge had misdirected the jury on the question of consent), the court accepted that the transmission of HIV could, in certain circumstances, amount to a criminal offence. A similar conclusion had already been reached in Scotland in 2001 (where a different system of criminal law applies), when Stephen Kelly was convicted of having 'recklessly injured' his former partner by infecting her with HIV.

This section is intended to briefly outline the circumstances in which the transmission of HIV might amount to a criminal offence.

It should be stressed at the outset that prosecutions for the transmission of HIV are likely to be very rare. There have been none in Scotland since Stephen Kelly's conviction in 2001, although there have been two further prosecutions in England following on from the Dica case. All the prosecutions to date appear to have involved allegations of deception on the part of the persons prosecuted, such as a false claim that they had tested negative for HIV, rather than simply a failure by a person to disclose his or her HIV-positive status.

The offence is not, it should be noted, limited to HIV, but might extend to any other sexually transmitted infection which could be considered to amount to "grievous bodily harm".

The "state of mind" required for the offence

There is no question of any person being liable for a criminal offence simply because they have transmitted HIV to another person. To be guilty of any serious criminal offence, a person must have acted with a culpable state of mind — which lawyers refer to as mens rea. The mens rea required for the offence of inflicting grievous bodily harm is intention or recklessness. In other words, for a conviction, it would be necessary to show that the defendant intended to infect the other party with HIV, or that they were reckless as to this possibility — that is, that the defendant was aware of the risk of infection. This would also be necessary in Scotland for the offence of "reckless injury" of which Stephen Kelly was convicted.

It is theoretically possible, therefore, that a person could be guilty of this offence even if they had not received a positive result from an HIV test. It would, however, be necessary to show that they were aware of a significant risk that they might be HIV-positive — for example, if they had previously been regularly engaged in unprotected intercourse with a person or persons whom they knew to be HIV-positive. While a prosecution in such a case would be unlikely, it should be made clear that avoiding taking an HIV test does not provide immunity from criminal prosecution. One of the English prosecutions to date involved a man who had never taken an HIV test, but had been told by his wife that she had tested positive for HIV shortly before he embarked on a relationship with another woman.

What is the effect of consent?

In quashing Mohammed Dica's convictions, the Court of Appeal ruled that, where a person chooses to consent to the risk of HIV transmission (that is, they know that their sexual partner is HIV-positive and choose to have unprotected intercourse regardless of this fact), then that will be a valid defence to a criminal prosecution. This would not, however, apply in the unlikely event that the consenting party had actually wanted to become infected with HIV (and the other party had intended this to happen). It is thought that the Scottish courts would take the same view.

What if condoms are used, or high-risk activities avoided?

What is the situation if a person who is HIV-positive does not disclose this fact to their sexual partner, but uses condoms, and HIV is nevertheless transmitted? In the Dica case, the Court of Appeal suggested that the use of condoms might mean that the HIV-positive person could not be said to have acted "recklessly", and so therefore would not have the state of mind required for the offence. Similarly, if the parties refrain from high-risk sexual activities, again, "recklessness" would not be present. A problem does arise, however, in relation to unprotected oral sex, which is not normally considered high-risk but which does present a more than negligible risk. It is thought that it would not be caught by the criminal law, but the exact position is unclear.

What if transmission does not occur?

In England and Wales, if an HIV-positive person has unprotected sexual intercourse without disclosing their serostatus, but the other party does not become infected, then a prosecution would be very unlikely. It is possible that there could be a prosecution for an attempt to inflict grievous bodily harm in such a case, but the prosecutor would have to show that the defendant actually intended to transmit the disease. It would not be enough to show that the positive person was simply reckless as to the possibility of the disease being transmitted. In Scotland, however, it is at least theoretically possible that there could be a prosecution for "reckless endangerment" in the absence of actual transmission.

A duty to disclose?

Because consent is a valid defence, it seems fair to say that the Dica case effectively places a legal duty on HIV-positive persons to disclose their HIV-status before engaging in high-risk sexual activities.

Immigration and asylum law

Introduction

UK immigration law is governed by the Immigration Act 1971. This has since been amended by subsequent pieces of legislation, particularly the Nationality, Immigration and Asylum Act 2002. More specific regulations are contained in the Immigration Rules, which are made by the Home Secretary and laid before Parliament.

This section provides a brief overview of immigration and asylum law as it affects people with HIV. It is, however, in no way a comprehensive statement of the law and is no substitute for specialist advice. Immigration law is complex, changes frequently and it can be important to meet deadlines and follow correct procedures in order to preserve your legal rights. For that reason, anyone facing a problem concerned with this area of the law should seek proper advice at the earliest possible opportunity.

The relevance of being HIV-positive

Neither the legislation nor the Immigration Rules specifically mention HIV. The UK has not adopted a ban on persons with HIV entering the United Kingdom, unlike a small number of other countries (including, most significantly, the USA). HIV-positive status may nevertheless be relevant to asylum and immigration decisions, depending on the type of decision concerned and the situation of the individual concerned. It is essential here to distinguish between different categories of persons. There are, essentially, two questions: first, can being HIV-positive or having been diagnosed with AIDS be a barrier to entering the UK? And secondly, where a person is already in the UK, can being HIV-positive or diagnosed with AIDS be a reason which justifies continuing to remain in the UK when that individual would otherwise be required to leave?

People not subject to UK immigration law

Most obviously, British citizens are not subject to immigration law. Nor are citizens of other states within the European Economic Area (EEA), who have specific rights of entry to the UK. Certain Commonwealth citizens also have a "right of abode" in the UK. For these persons, being HIV-positive should not affect entry into the UK.

Any other person, however, requires leave to enter the UK.

Leave to enter the UK and HIV-positive status

Where a person requires leave to enter, the UK's current (and long-standing) policy is that the fact that a person is HIV-positive, or has AIDS, is not in itself a ground for refusing leave to enter the UK. (Leave may, of course, still be refused if that person does not otherwise qualify for leave under the Rules.) However, the effect which a medical condition may have on a person's ability to support himself or herself is a factor which the Immigration Officer may take into account in deciding whether to grant leave to enter.

A person who intends to remain in the UK for more than six months should normally be referred to the Medical Inspector for examination, and the inspector will be expected to estimate the cost of any treatment which may be required so that this can be considered by the Immigration Officer.

Entering the UK for medical treatment

A person may seek leave to enter or remain in the UK in order to
receive private medical treatment. In particular, it will be
necessary for such a person to show that he or she has sufficient
funds to meet the costs of treatment. It is also necessary that the
applicant "can show, if required to do so, that any proposed
course of treatment is of finite duration". It would not, therefore,
normally be possible to use these provisions to seek entry to the
UK for ongoing HIV or AIDS treatment, although they could, for
example, apply for leave to enter to seek treatment for an HIV-
related illness. Leave to enter for private medical treatment will,
in practice, only be a realistic option for the relatively wealthy.
NHS treatment is not automatically free for those from overseas.

Can HIV be a ground for remaining in the UK?

Where a person is entitled to apply for leave to remain on
grounds unrelated to their HIV-positive status, then the same
principle as noted earlier applies: the fact that someone is HIV-
positive or has AIDS is not in itself a basis for refusing that
application.

However, there may be cases where a person has no other grounds
to remain in the UK, but wishes to seek discretionary leave to
remain on the basis that they will not receive adequate medical
treatment in their home country.

Such applications may be bolstered by reference to the European
Convention on Human Rights, article 3 of which provides that
"no one shall be subjected to torture or to inhuman or degrading
treatment or punishment". In this context, reference is often
made to the decision of the European Court of Human Rights in
the case D v United Kingdom (1997) 24 EHRR 423. In that
case, D was serving a period of imprisonment in the UK for a
drug related offence. While he was in prison, he was diagnosed as
being HIV-positive and suffering from AIDS. After his release,
the government proposed to return him to his home country, St
Kitts. The European Court noted that D was very close to death,
that the care available for him in St Kitts would be inadequate,
and that his removal would expose him to a real risk of dying

under most distressing circumstances. It would, therefore, potentially amount to inhuman treatment under article 3, meaning that the UK government could not return him to St Kitts as intended.

Further reading

James Chalmers, 'Criminalising HIV Infection,' *AIDS Treatment Update* 131.

Work

Introduction

The 1996 edition of *Living with HIV and AIDS* contained hardly any information on working if you are HIV-positive. Until effective anti-HIV treatment became available, shortly after the last edition of this book was published, HIV services were largely geared towards helping people claim their state benefits and managing retirement from work on the basis of ill health.

It's perhaps an indication of just how successful anti-HIV treatment can be that many people with HIV are now either remaining in the workplace or thinking about returning to work or study.

Work can have many advantages, including stimulation, enjoyment, a sense of accomplishment, company and friendship – and a regular financial income.

There can, however, be some very real difficulties returning to work after having a prolonged period of time off due to illness. There's also a chance that you might encounter some difficulties in the workplace related to your HIV infection.

Going back to work

An early, and important decision you'll need to make is what workdo you wish to do?

You might want to pick up where you left off. However, particularly if it's a long time since you were last employed, starting again where you left off might not be an option.

Alternatively, you might want to use your return to work as an opportunity to change direction and enter a new line of work.

For some people with HIV, it's not a question of "returning" to work, but of entering the workplace for the first time.

Whatever situation you're in, there's a good chance you'll need some training to help you prepare, both practically and mentally, for work.

Training

If you want to gain new skills or experience, you could perhaps do some voluntary work, enroll in a course, or register on a training scheme.

Volunteering can provide an opportunity to gain new skills and at the same time gain a familiarity with working conditions. The routine of volunteering can also help simulate the routine of working, and if you are volunteering in an area similar to the one in which you'd like to work, it can provide an opportunity to discover if this really is something you'd like to do.

Many people find that volunteering helps boost their self-confidence and acts as a useful bridge back to work.

Studying

To gain employment in your area of interest, it might be necessary to gain specific skills or a qualification. Colleges and universities around the country have part-time study opportunities for adults, ranging from open access courses with no entry requirements to higher degrees.

As well as equipping you with skills and qualifications, studying can help focus your attention on what job or career you'd like to undertake, and build your confidence.

Help for applying for jobs

Local job centres and some HIV organisations can help you develop or enhance your job application and interview skills.

The impact of returning to work or study

If you left work a number of years ago, or have never worked, the prospect of getting a job can be daunting. Your confidence might be low, you might feel left behind or deskilled. Although you may be able to go straight into full-time employment, a more realistic plan might be to undertake some part-time work, either paid or voluntary, or study, and find a working balance that suits you.

The impact that working or studying can have on your benefits can be a real worry. Many people with HIV have reported being in a "benefits trap". If you qualify for the maximum rate of benefits, you might actually be financially worse off if you return to work, unless the job is very well paid.

You might also be deterred from thinking about work or study because you are uncertain about how long you'll remain healthy, or are worried that working might damage your health.

Working with HIV

Disclosure

Unless you're working in certain healthcare professions, there's absolutely no requirement for you to tell your employer that you're HIV-positive.

Nevertheless, you may choose to tell your employer in the hope that this will lead to a more supportive working environment. However, you may prefer to keep information about your health confidential in order to avoid discrimination or having to deal with colleagues' attitudes towards HIV.

If you need time off because of illness or for hospital appointments think about how you are going to explain this without disclosing your HIV status.

HIV testing

There's no law to stop an employer asking for an HIV test as part of a company medical for new employees. However, they've no right to see the result of the test result without your consent.

The only way an employer can ask an existing employee to take an HIV test is if the initial terms and conditions of a job said that this would be the case.

Employment rights

The Disability Discrimination Act provides important workplace protection to people with HIV from the moment of their HIV diagnosis. These rights are on top of those provided by other legislation.

Basically, it is unlawful for an employer with 15 or more employees to:

• Discriminate against an HIV-positive person in recruitment and selection unless this can be 'justified'.

• Give an HIV-positive person less favourable treatment (including access to promotion, training and transfers, as well as dismissal and selection for redundancy) unless this can be 'justified'.

• Fail to make 'reasonable' adjustments to the work environment to enable an HIV-positive person to work.

Can my employer sack me because I'm ill due to HIV?

UK Government guidelines in the booklet *AIDS and the Workplace* state that:

"HIV infection alone does not affect people's ability to do their job until they develop illnesses that make them unfit... If they later become ill, they should be treated like anyone else with a life-threatening illness. Only if their illness affects their ability to do the job should their employer seek medical advice."

The only way this advice will have changed since the Disability Discrimination Act is that the employer must have considered reasonable adjustments before dismissing you as a result of HIV-related illness.

If you are dismissed because you are unable to do the job, the employer must have sufficient evidence upon which to base that decision. This involves, preferably, both a report from the employee's doctor and an examination by a doctor on behalf of the employer.

If you are physically unable to carry out your contractual job, then the employer should consider the possibility of a move to different duties. The likelihood of there being suitable alternative employment will depend largely on the size of the firm involved. Furthermore, there is no duty for the employer to create alternative employment.

Seek legal advice if your employer is causing you difficulties in relation to time off for sickness.

Further reading

A good place to start is the UKC's "Into work guide" which can be accessed on their website www.ukcoalition.org. A printed copy of the guide can be obtained by calling 020 7564 2180.

'Employment,' in NAM's *AIDS Reference Manual* (last updated in June 2003).

Finding information

Introduction

There are many organisations around the UK offering services and information to people with HIV.

NAM publishes the *UK AIDS Directory* every year. It includes information on HIV clinics and services providers throughout the UK. You can also search for HIV clinics on NAM's website www.aidsmap.com.

There have been a lot of changes in the HIV voluntary sector, with many organisations either merging with other HIV charities or closing altogether.

To find out what HIV services are available near you, a good place to start would be to call one of the national helplines listed below or talk to one of the professionals you are currently receiving HIV services from.

The quality of HIV information on the internet ranges from excellent to mad, bad, and dangerous to know. Details of a few key sites are listed below.

National Helplines

National Drugs Helpline
0800 776 600 (freephone)

Every day 24 hours

National free helpline offering advice, information and referrals on all drug issues including HIV and AIDS.

National Sexual Health Helpline

0800 567 123 (freephone)

Every day 24 hours

National telephone helpline answering calls on all aspects of sexual health including HIV.

NHS Direct

0845 4647 (calls charged at local rate)

Every day 24 hours

www.nhsdirect.nhs.uk

NHS Direct provides a 24 hour nurse advice and health information service, providing confidential information on what to do if you are feeling ill, general information on health conditions, local health services such as GPs and late night chemists, and support and self help groups.

THT Direct

0845 1221 200 (calls charged at local rate)

Mon – Fri   10am – 10pm

Sat – Sun   12noon – 6pm

www.tht.org.uk

A gateway to HIV information, services and support provided by the Terrence Higgins Trust (THT), the largest HIV charity in the UK. THT provide extensive published information and a wide range of support and advocacy services.

THT currently offers services in London, Bath, Birmingham, Brighton, Bristol, Cardiff, Coventry, Eastboure, Essex, Leeds, Oxford, Surrey, Swansea, Swindon and Wolverhampton. Details of the services available at each centre and how to access them can be obtained from THT direct.

i-Base Treatment Information Phoneline
0808 800 6013 (freephone)

Mon – Weds   12noon – 4pm

www.i-base.org

Phone line providing confidential information on HIV treatment.

Key self-help, advocacy and specialist groups

African HIV Policy Network (AHPN)
New City Cloisters
196 Old Street
London EC1V PFR
020 7017 8912
info@ahpn.org
www.ahpn.org

The African HIV Policy Network (AHPN) is an umbrella
organisation which represents African community groups
addressing HIV/AIDS and sexual health throughout the UK.

GMFA
Unit 43 Eurolink Centre
49 Effra Road
London SW2 1BZ
020 7738 7140
gmfa@gmfa.org.uk
www.metromate.org.uk

GMFA (Gay Men Fighting AIDS) is is a London-based, volunteer-
led gay men's health organisation. Volunteers are supported and
trained to develop and execute health interventions for gay men.
GMFA's HIV prevention interventions include workshops, press
adverts, a newsletter and this website. Their interventions to
improve the health of HIV positive gay men include press work

and workshops. GMFA's general health work includes smoking cessation workshops.

The Haemophilia Society

3rd Floor

Chesterfield House

385 Euston Road

London NW1 3AU

020 7380 0600

0800 018 6068 (freephone helpline)

Mon-Fri   9am – 5pm

info@haemophilia.org.uk

www.haemophilia.org.uk

The Society is involved in providing advocacy, information, support and advice to all those living with haemophilia and other blood clotting disorders. The Society also supports those with blood clotting disorders and viral hepatitis as a result of their NHS treatment with infected blood products.

Mainliners

38-40 Kennington Park Road

London SE11 4RS

020 7582 6999

020 7582 5226 (helpline)

Mon-Fri   10am-6pm

admin@mainliners.org.uk

Mainliners works with former and current injecting drug users and commercial sex workers affected by and infected with HIV and/or hepatitis.

NAZ Project

Palingswick House (annex)

241 King St

London W6 9LP

020 8741 1879

naz@naz.org.uk

www.naz.org.uk

Naz Project London provides sexual health and HIV prevention and support services to South Asian, Middle Eastern, North African, Horn of African and Latin American Communities.

Naz aims to educate and empower communities to face up to the challenges of sexual health and the AIDS pandemic, and to mobilise the support networks that exist for people living with HIV/AIDS.

Positively Women

347-349 City Road

London EC1V 1LR

020 7713 0444

info@positivelywomen.org.uk

www.positivelywomen.org.uk

A national charity working to life of women and families affected by HIV.

UK Coalition of People Living with HIV and AIDS (UKC)

250 Kennington Lane

London SE11 5RD

020 7564 2180

reception@ukcoalition.org

www.ukcoalition.org

UKC is a group of people living with HIV and AIDS, campaigning, researching and providing services by and for people with HIV. Publishers of *Positive Nation* the UK's HIV and sexual health magazine.

Websites

AEGIS

www.aegis.com

The most extensive collection of links on AIDS, with searchable electronic versions of many newsletters and a vast catalogue of news stories, plus discussion forums.

AIDS

www.aidsonline.com

An influential medical journal sponsored by the International AIDS Society, with free access to abstracts, which provide a summary of the key findings of research. Full text access only available to subscribers.

aidsmap.com

www.aidsmap.com

NAM's website. On this site you can find more original, daily news on developments in the world of HIV than any other HIV website. The site also includes completely searchable databases of HIV treatment and care, worldwide HIV organisation listings, and one of the most comprehensive ranges of patient information available on the web.

American Foundation for AIDS Research (AMFAR)

www.amfar.org

A good searchable treatment database excellent news and analysis and a nice simple design.

Clinical Care Options for HIV

www.clinicaloptions.com/hiv

A site targeted at HIV medical professionals.

HIVandHepatitis.com
www.hivandhepatitis.com

This site concentrates on news and conference reports, largely targeted at medical professionals.

HIVInsite
www.hivinsite.com

The electronic version of the AIDS Knowledge Base, a textbook developed by physicians at San Francisco General Hospital. The site also contains databases on trials, drug interactions and side effects, as well as news stories and a library of reports on prevention issues.

International AIDS Society
www.ias.se

Website of the International AIDS Society which includes daily news. The site also makes available abstracts of conferences organised by the International AIDS Society including the International AIDS Conference.

Medscape
www.medscape.com/hiv-aidshome

Another site designed to provide doctors with continuing medical education on HIV. The site also provides daily news and conference coverage.

The Body
www.thebody.com

An extensive collection of articles from HIV newsletters and other publications around the world, and an exclusive "Ask the Experts" forum for you to put questions to the leading doctors.

UNAIDS
www.unaids.com

United Nations AIDS Programme – information about the activities of the programme, access to policy documents and records of UNAIDS-sponsored interventions; statistics on the global epidemic.

Index

S

Other information available from NAM

Whether you are recently diagnosed, starting or changing treatment, or have been on treatment for a long time, NAM produces a range of information resources to support you in the choices you make about your health and treatment options.

Monthly Newsletter

AIDS Treatment Update is a monthly newsletter, written to support you in the decisions you make about living healthily with HIV. It keeps you up to date with the latest treatment news, and each month contains feature articles looking at different issues related to living well with HIV.

Monthly Factsheets

Our one page factsheets provide basic overviews on a wide range of topics related to your health and HIV. We publish a new factsheet each month.

Information booklets

This series of 14 booklets provides plain English introductory guides to key treatment topics.

www.aidsmap.com

Visit our website, aidsmap.com, for instant access to:
- a fully searchable treatments database
- a complete list of sexual health clinics in the UK
- daily news stories and conference reporting from around the world
- online access to all the resources listed above

To order copies of any of these resources please return the form opposite or contact NAM by email or telephone:
NAM, Freepost LON17995, London SW9 6BR
tel 020 7840 0050
email info@nam.org.uk

order form

name

address

email

signature

AIDS Treatment Update
Please set up my free* subscription to AIDS Treatment Update ☐
Please circle the format you require: paper / email(pdf) / audio tape

NAM factsheets
Please set up my free* subscription to the monthly factsheets ☐
Please send me factsheets on the following:
☐Anti-HIV drugs, ☐Anti-HIV therapy, ☐Immune system,
☐Hepatitis, ☐Healthy Living, ☐Lipodystrophy,
☐Opportunistic Infections/Health Problems, ☐Rcreational Drugs,
☐Reproductive Health, ☐Services and Sources of Information,
☐Sexual Health, ☐Side Effects

Please circle the format you require: paper / email (pdf)

Information Booklets
Please send me the following free* booklets
☐ Adherence, ☐Anti HIV Drugs, ☐Children and HIV, ☐Clinical Trials,
☐Glossary, ☐HIV & Children, ☐HIV & Hepatitis, ☐HIV & Sex,
☐HIV & TB, ☐HIV Therapy,☐HIV & Women, ☐Lipodystrophy,
☐Nutrition, ☐Resistance, ☐Viral Load & CD4

How do we store your details? Your address details are stored by NAM in a password-protected database. Your details will not be passed on to any third party.

NAM publishes a range of information resources on HIV and AIDS. Please tick this box if you would not like to be added to our mailing list ☐

NAM occasionally undertakes fundraising campaigns to help support our work. Please tick this box if you would not like to receive information about them. ☐

*We are unable to provide these resources free to professionals and organisations. Please contact NAM for prices.